Diabetic

Heal Thyself

NATURALLY

a SimpleGuy Solutions^{SM}

TO CONTROLLING TYPE 2 DIABETES *without* Rx MEDICATIONS

The Plan that dropped my blood sugar numbers from 341 to 113—without Rx medicine—in less than four months!

Cover Design by LifeSource Creations
Cover Graphic by ©iStock.com/ayzek
Published by LifeSource Creations/SimpleGuy Solutions[sm]
www.simpleguysolutions.com
Title: Diabetic Heal Thyself Naturally/SimpleGuy Solutions
ISBN: 978-0-9908762-8-1

Table of Contents

Introduction

> *"You are* ***not*** *paying attention! You don't realize how serious this is," he said. "You should have been admitted to the hospital and put on insulin immediately until your blood sugar goes down."*

These were the sobering words of a close doctor friend when he found out I was not yet on the diabetic medicine that had been prescribed for me. In a sense, he was right. We just didn't realize it at the time. It got even worse a few days later.

I was having lunch with another friend who had some gift cards he had received at Christmas and wanted to take me out to a nice Cajun restaurant for lunch. The key word to describe our lunch that day was *fried*: fried fish, French fries and fried hushpuppies. A nutritionist would describe it as carbs, carbs, carbs, with a dash of protein. I did thoroughly enjoy the meal! When it was over, I can't say that I felt badly—but I did feel that maybe I had overdone it. My wife suggested I test my blood sugar. Since we had just purchased our new blood glucose (sugar) testing "kit," I agreed. It registered 421 mg/dl! That is not a misprint—**421** mg/dl. That number immediately got our attention.

At that point, we did not know much about diabetes, but we had heard that if your blood sugar number gets to 600 mg/dl, you are in the danger zone and can go into a diabetic coma. We weren't interested in dealing with that, so our journey into the world of diabetes got very intense—very fast!

I want to interject here that the reason I am writing this little book is because, as of this morning, about 4 months later, my blood glucose/sugar reading was 106 mg/dl—and we never took the medicine, even for a short time.

This is the story of how we accomplished that, as well as some of the things we came to understand along the way (like the reality that the mainstream medical approach to diabetes **seems** to be designed to **keep** you on the medicine for the rest of your life!). It does ***not*** have to be that way. If you are reading this book, I assume you want to know how we did it. This is our story.

[Note: In this book, we will use the terms, blood ***glucose*** and blood ***sugar,*** interchangeably. Blood sugar is the more common layman's term, blood glucose is the more technical/medical term. They refer to the same thing. It is describing the amount of sugar/glucose in the blood at any given time.]

The art of healing comes from nature, **not** *from the physician. Therefore, the physician must start from nature, with an open mind.*

– Paracelsus (Father of Toxicology)

Chapter 1

We Were Not Trying To Be Difficult...Really!

That really is the truth. I had just received the results back from the blood tests my doctor had taken a few days before. We talked with the doctor's office, and were informed that the doctor wanted to start me on insulin immediately. My A1c Hemoglobin reading showed that my blood glucose level was over 13.4 (this meant my blood glucose/sugar level was averaging about 321 mg/dl over a 90-day period. Since anything over 125 mg/dl is considered to be in the "diabetic" range, in his words, it was totally out of control. Medicine (i.e., insulin) was the answer.

I have a brother who also was diagnosed with diabetes (as was my father, so it's in the family DNA), and he has been on diabetic medicine (Metformin) for several years. Knowing this, I asked my doctor if we could start with Metformin first instead of going right on insulin.

He agreed, but said that we should be prepared, that it often takes more than one medication to keep blood sugar under control if one chooses not to take insulin.

By the way, you will find an Appendix in the back of the book detailing how we have managed to control all of our medical costs for the last 15 years. If you feel that healthcare costs are simply consuming too much of your budget and would like to have a viable, economical alternative which allows you total control of which doctors and hospitals treat you, this program will interest you. If you still have questions, send an email to *equity1st@yahoo.com* and put "CHM Healthcare" in the subject, and we will send you more info.

My wife and I are covered for all major medical expenses up to at least $125,000 per incident for about $170/month. No, that is not a misprint—and it is the total cost per month, not per person. It is possible (and for a very small add-on program, this number increases to $1,000,000). We've been on it for over 10 years, have referred many friends, and never had any problems. It works. It was given a specific exemption in the ObamaCare law, so it fulfilled all legal healthcare requirements under that law. If you need to reduce your healthcare costs, it is definitely worth a serious look.

Back to my story.

The doctor ordered the Rx *Metformin* medicine for me. (By the way, my doctor was a VA [U.S. Department of Veterans Affairs] doctor. I am a Vietnam veteran, but had only served four years on active duty. I knew that those who had served 20 or more years had lifetime access to VA medical services, but I had no idea that for a very nominal fee, I could have access also.)

Fortunately, because of the cost-sharing program I describe in the Appendix, I don't have to rely solely on him for final decisions regarding any serious major illnesses or treatments; still I think he's a pretty good doctor. I know some have had problems with the VA, but I have not. He had been urging me for over a year to address my blood sugar levels when they were in the 125–130 mg/dl range—a range he rightly considered "borderline" diabetic. Like so many of us though, sometimes it's hard to get our attention.

To his credit, he urged that we establish a regimen that focused on diet and exercise. So, he wasn't one to quickly jump and put me on drugs. I appreciated that. I simply did ***not*** take the warnings about my potential blood sugar problems seriously enough. Now I had no choice.

Why Are We Writing This Book?

We believe there are a lot of people like us who would rather *not* go down the path of taking diabetic medicine for the rest of their lives. And, make no mistake about it, once you go down that path, it is *very* difficult to get off it. Why? Because the people who could help you the most are making money if you stay on the medicine. It's simply not in their best economic interest to help you get off the medication.

It is also true that much of mainstream medicine operates (even if they won't admit it) on the premise that if you can mitigate (i.e., lessen or mask) the symptoms long enough, the body will eventually heal itself.

Did you get that? You might want to read that again. To us, that's just part of the miracle of creation. The body **is**, in fact, designed to heal itself! And most of the time it does, if you give it what it needs.

We know and agree that there are times when drastic measures are needed to protect life. But we also believe that God designed the body so that if we treat it right, when illness strikes, it can often heal itself if given the right "tools." Sometimes, prescription medicine *is* what you need, but sometimes there is an alternative. But be forewarned, prescription medicine often has serious downsides.

In this case, diabetic medicine does not lead to the potential option of the body healing itself. It is one of those remedies that leads to "maintenance." In other words, once you start it and get the symptoms under control, you have to stay with it. We didn't want to go that way if we could avoid it. So, we were pretty much on our own. Adding to the problem was the fact that there wasn't much information or encouragement readily available to tell us how we could do that.

It was my wife (trusting God for wisdom) who undertook the task of searching the Internet for weeks, and who deserves all the credit for tracking down leads and suggestions of things which might aid us in the quest to get control of this disease. In the end, we were forced to assemble all the pieces ourselves. But at least the pieces were out there.

Is There a *Cure?*

Please note, we **never** use the word *cure* in this book. The National Library of Medicine states, *"Diabetes is a lifelong disease and there is no cure."*[1] We believe it's best to accept that diagnosis in the same way we accept that an addict can never claim to be *cured*. But he can *recover*, and that recovery can allow him or her to lead a relatively normal life, as long as he avoids the things that caused the problem in the first place.

In our estimation, diabetes can be considered as a form of addiction. Think of it as a sugar addiction; you likely got where you are because you indulged in too much of the *quick high* sugar treats, the unhealthy fats, and the over-abundance of carbohydrates, (i.e., things that often quickly turn to sugar)

Some folks may argue, *"I wasn't that bad; I tried to eat healthy!"* This may be true, but most of us are simply not aware of how much things like HFCS (high fructose corn syrup) permeates our packaged groceries. Once you start looking at labels, you will begin to shake your head in disbelief.

It is literally everywhere! What food suppliers have realized is that Americans will eat almost anything—if it is sweet enough. This is why almost ***100 million Americans*** are either already diagnosed as diabetic or on the verge of becoming one. It is no exaggeration to call this a national epidemic.

You have to recognize this and replace these foods with a specially designed and targeted *balance* of foods which will enable the body to perform the way it was designed to perform. You can't keep on doing what you have been doing and expect to see different results. You have to change some things if you want different results. And, you can do it.

The reason we are writing this book is to share the things we have uncovered and the regimen that we discovered and adopted that enabled us to bring my blood sugar numbers from over 340 mg/dl down to 110–115 mg/dl in just 3 months—and without medication of any sort.

It ***is*** possible. And, yes, you **will** have to make some lifestyle changes, and it **will** require commitment—seriously diligent commitment—for at least a few months until you have achieved your desired goal and stabilized there. Once you are in the maintenance phase, you may indulge yourself once in a while—within limits. The key is you will know how to recover quickly. That is really important!

If you are going to regain control of your blood sugar, you need a plan—a plan to which you are willing to commit.

The *first* phase of this plan is to allow at least three to four months to achieve your goal. We have to remember that none of us got into this condition overnight, and we can't solve the problem overnight.

Once you make the commitment to set yourself on this regimen for three–four months, you need to stay on it *religiously.* Why? So your body (more specifically your pancreas) can begin to heal. It's been abused for a long time. It needs to heal and this will take time, rest, and healthy nutrition.

We're also going to share some critical, nutritional supplement suggestions that we uncovered in our research efforts. We believe these are *crucial* to your success, and we'll give you options for where to find the best bargains on them as well. There are usually no bargains in the health food store—but there are some great, economical options, especially online.

We will also share our diet and exercise regimen with you—along with some recipes that will (we hope!) really brighten up your experience. As you might know, diabetics are often viewed as having to be on a *bland* diet. True or false?

We have **not** found that to be true at all (unless you believe life is bland without cokes and potato chips, and that everything laden with high fructose corn syrup is an essential of life!). Some things will be different, to be sure, but once you have decided to change your ways, you will likely find lots of things getting better; you may find you end up living longer, too!

The Discovery of My Disease was a "Fluke"

It was kind of a fluke that we discovered I had a serious problem to begin with. It was just after the Christmas/New Year's holiday season had ended. I was putting on some pants and realized they seemed awfully loose. We all know that's *not* usually the problem after those holidays, right? That's what I thought as well. I'm not one who is constantly checking the scales, so I had to check it. I had lost about 15 pounds—without trying.

At my age (60+), losing weight without trying is usually **not** a good sign. Things like pancreatic cancer come to mind as the potential problem. But whatever the cause, it was best to find out ASAP.

I was overdue for my semi-annual doctor visit anyway, so now I was motivated to get my blood work done to see if I could figure out what was going on. The tests revealed that it **was** a pancreatic problem; thankfully, it was **not** pancreatic cancer.

The diagnosis was quick and definitive:

You are now a diabetic.

But what does that *really* mean? Let's think about that.

[Note: It is a medical fact of life that some Rx medicines which are prescribed to treat various diseases (especially statin drugs which attempt to reduce cholesterol to address cardiovascular disease issues) often push pre-diabetic persons into the full-blown diabetic category. In Chapter 6 we address why we believe that inflammation (not cholesterol) is the real problem behind the dramatic rise in heart disease. However, this book is primarily intended to help those whose diabetic challenges can be met with diet and exercise, not those caused by Rx drugs.]

Chapter 2

What's Really Wrong with You?

> There is one consolation in being sick; and that is the possibility that you may recover to a better state than you were ever in before.
>
> —Henry David Thoreau

Honestly, I did not know. I had heard somewhere that diabetes was a blood sugar problem—but what does that mean anyway? I was clueless. Another challenge that made the problem even worse was that I basically felt fine! Diseases without visible or even painful symptoms can be deadly. Why? As we all know, we tend to ignore them.

I knew I did not have the stamina I used to have, but that could have been caused by any number of things, including just getting older. I knew bright lights hurt my eyes late at night, but I was also tired by then. There just wasn't anything I could point to that drove me to find out what the problem was. The weight loss did the trick.

Like most folks, I had been trying to lose ten pounds (or more!) for several years (sound familiar?). Nothing seemed to work. When I would try to cut back on my eating, I felt horrible (the bloated feeling was awful). Even more exercise didn't seem to make a difference. I really had stopped trying. So, for me to see 12–13 pounds disappear without trying was very suspicious. I knew that meant something was happening, but it probably wasn't good. That's when we got the blood work done and discovered the real problem. Here's the crash course:

What we learned was this: Diabetes is a **pancreas** problem.

What does the **pancreas** do? It's an organ that produces **insulin**.

What is **insulin**? It's a hormone, like estrogen or testosterone.

What does it do? **Insulin** regulates sugar in the bloodstream.

How does it do that? It enables the sugar in the bloodstream to be absorbed by the cells in your muscles, fat, and liver. It's used to give your body energy to function.

If there is excess **glucose** (sugar) in the blood, it stimulates the muscles and liver to store it. When the sugar is stored like this, instead of glucose, it is called **glycogen**. This whole process is designed to give your body the energy it needs to function—as well as a ready reserve if it's needed.

To be clear, as you surely can tell, what I am giving you is my best effort to translate what the medical professionals say about this into *layman's terms*. I am neither a scientist nor am I a medical professional. I am just a diligent student. I have been around the alternative health world for many years and believe God has created this world in such a way that all the answers to our most common health problems are right here on earth, if we only know how to find and use them.

Interestingly, many pharmaceutical products started as nothing more than natural products which have been researched and analyzed to determine the *active* ingredient (the essential thing that makes it effective) in the chemical compounds. Then they artificially, chemically re-create these active ingredients. And of course, this chemical *creation* is then patented and sold to us for enormous profits.

According to endocrineweb.com:

> "Insulin is a hormone made by the pancreas that allows your body to use sugar (glucose) from carbohydrates in the food that you eat for energy or to store glucose for future use. Insulin helps keeps your blood sugar level from getting too high (hyperglycemia) or too low (hypoglycemia).
>
> "The cells in your body need sugar for energy. However, sugar cannot go into most of your cells directly. After you eat food and your blood sugar level rises, cells in your pancreas (known as beta cells) are signaled to release insulin into your bloodstream.
>
> "Insulin then attaches to and signals cells to absorb

> sugar from the bloodstream. Insulin is often described as a "key" which unlocks the cell door to allow sugar to enter the cell and be used for energy."[1]

When Do You Know You Have a Problem?

You have a problem when your pancreas either produces no insulin (type 1 diabetes) or has been so exhausted that it is overwhelmed and can no longer effectively aid in the removal of the sugar from the bloodstream (type 2 diabetes). This condition is often called, pre-diabetes or *insulin resistance* (technically this isn't type 2, but it's usually considered a "pit stop" on the way to full-blown diabetes). The degree of impairment is normally reflected in your blood glucose test numbers.

If you truly have type 1 diabetes (which usually means your pancreas is producing no insulin at all), you will likely have no alternative but to take insulin. Your healthcare professional will instruct you on how to deal with this. Your diet and exercise regimen will have an important part in determining just how much insulin you need to take, but insulin will be essential. But this is not an area to go "rogue" on. Listen to your doctor!

If you have diabetes, or especially if you have pre-diabetic insulin resistance, the regimen we will share can greatly help you.

Type 2 diabetes means that your pancreas is still producing some insulin (but not enough to handle the carbohydrate load with which you may be burdening it through poor eating habits).

In the case of pre-diabetes caused by insulin resistance there is some impairment, i.e., *resistance*, occurring in the metabolic process which would normally allow the blood sugar to be transferred from the bloodstream into the cells by the insulin hormones so that it can provide energy for the body's various functions.

The good news is that either cause may be dealt with by using the same restorative regimen we describe in this book.

What Is Your Real Goal?

This may seem like a foolish question at first, but stop and think about it. *Understanding* what your real problem is can help focus your efforts to heal yourself, not just put on a medical "Band-Aid" to get by.

If your problem is an *exhausted* pancreas which isn't producing enough insulin to handle the burden you are putting on it, what are you accomplishing if you just give the body more insulin? Are you solving the problem? No. You are removing the excess blood sugar, but the pancreas is *still* exhausted. You haven't dealt with the core problem at all. Isn't your ultimate goal to get your pancreas back to true health? Of course it is, or you wouldn't be reading this book.

If your problem is *insulin resistance*, it means that your cells are not readily absorbing the sugar/glucose from the blood. Why not? What is the real problem?

The answer most often given is *metabolic syndrome*. What does that mean? When you see the word *syndrome* being used to describe some malady, it is usually medical code for "we really don't know what causes this malfunction, so we call it a

syndrome. We see it a lot—so we can't ignore it—but we really have no clue what causes it."

Unfortunately, the doctor will often feel pressured to prescribe some generic, broad spectrum antibiotic (rather than tell you, "We need to watch this and see if something more develops so we know what we are dealing with and can treat it properly."), just so you won't feel like you wasted your time coming to see the doctor.

While that may not be very comforting, at least it's honest! And to be fair, the problem often lies as much with our expectations of the doctor as it does with his treatment of us.

What do the "experts" know about people with metabolic syndrome?

They know that people who have it tend to have at least *two* things in common. **They have poor diets and they are overweight.** You know—typical Americans. We may chuckle at that, but the statistics relative to diabetics are not a joke. And most folks have no idea how serious this problem is. But you need to know because it's a BIG problem...for lots of us!

Here is a summary of some of the latest reports...

The Statistics

How many Americans have diabetes? According to the American Diabetes Association (ADA), as of 2012 (the latest available data), over **29 million** Americans have diabetes. That's a big number. But it gets worse; one out of four are not diagnosed…in other words, they don't even know they have it!

How many Americans have *prediabetes?* Are you sitting down? ***Over 86 million have it!*** And that number is going up at a rate of about 10% every two years in the most recent reports.

What is the difference between *diabetes* and *prediabetes?* Simply the number on the scale. If your blood glucose number is 100-125 mg/dl, they call it *prediabetes.*

If it's over 125 mg/dl, they call it *diabetes.* Unless something changes drastically, the statistics conclude that those who are now "labeled" as *pre-diabetic* will almost certainly have full-blown diabetes in 10 years or less. In other words unless you act now, it's not a matter of IF, but WHEN you will have it.

The drug companies love to hear that; they can hear the cash register ringing!

What is truly frightening is that *about 25% of these people have no clue that they have it.* Very often it will have few, if any, symptoms—until it has already begun to do damage—and it can do some real damage, both to your economic and physical health. The effects can be either life-changing or even life-threatening. The CDC (United States Centers for Disease Control) lists diabetes as the seventh leading cause of death in America.[2]

Some Sobering American Diabetic Association (ADA) Statistics

According to the ADA, minorities (African-Americans, Asian, Indian, and Hispanic) all tend to have a significantly higher risk of diabetes. While the rate among Caucasians is about 7.6%; among Asians, it's about 9%; among Hispanics, it's about

12.8%; among African-Americans, it's about 13.2%; and among American Indians, it runs almost 16%. These are serious numbers.[3]

The collateral damage from diabetes is real and needs to be taken seriously.

If you have diabetes, you have a 65% chance of having cholesterol problems, which means you could end up on that pharmaceutical treadmill as well. This can get expensive quickly...have you been to the ER lately?

In 2011 (most recent ADA data available), there were over 450,000 emergency room visits for either high or low blood sugar crises by diabetics.[4] Once you get on the medicine, if something really goes awry, you'll be heading for the ER...and those bills can cause heart attacks by themselves!

And speaking of heart attacks...

The death rates from CVD (cardiovascular disease) were 1.8x greater for diabetics than for non-diabetics. The chance of a diabetic having a stroke is 1.5x greater than non-diabetics.[5]

The collateral damage doesn't end there. About 25% of diabetics end up with eye problems that can cause partial or full blindness.[6]

Want to end up on a dialysis machine for the rest of your life? About 44% of all the kidney failures come from diabetic complications.

Want to keep both your feet on the ground? Of the 73,000 non-traumatic, lower limb amputations done in 2010, about 60% were the result of diabetic complications.[7]

In other words, it was not an injury that resulted in the amputations, it was a decision individuals made with their doctor after determining there was no other feasible alternative.

I know this is a lot of statistics, and obviously, these are serious statistics. But they represent more than that. They represent the real life experiences of folks just like you and me. But it's also true that, in the vast majority of cases, it does not have to be that way

There is a better way. So, let us show you how we did it. First, we want you to understand the Rx drug options—and why we did everything possible to avoid them.

Chapter 3

The Most Common Rx Drug Solution and Its Side-Effects

Disease is the biggest money-maker in our economy.
-John Tobe, Author

Why Were We So Concerned?

The first thing you must try to understand is that no one is really trying to **cure** your type 2 diabetes. We don't really comprehend that when the doctor writes out our first prescription. It normally does not dawn on us that what he is doing is prescribing a prescription drug to **control** it, not cure it. As far as the medical establishment is concerned, there is no cure. And they have no incentive to cure it. The real money is in selling you medicine for the rest of your life to control it. And that is BIG money.

This is not to disparage the physician at all. Once you reach the point where your body can no longer adequately process the sugar in your blood efficiently, the standard medical care is to recommend that you take a prescription (Rx) drug to lower the sugar in your blood to a more acceptable level (historically, somewhere in the 100-125 mg/dl range—and depending on whomever you talk to today, many believe that below 100 mg/dl is the best target).

The root idea is that by using the drug, you can continue to live a fairly normal life (Translation: You can continue to do the things that got you in trouble in the first place, but avoid some of the pain.) It sounds like a great option—almost like "you can have your cake and eat it, too." So why would we look for another way, a natural alternative, one that did not include the use of Rx drugs? Why do this?

The main reason is we felt the cure might be worse than the disease. (Please don't misunderstand me here. If I ever reach a point that I can no longer control my blood sugar naturally, then I would not hesitate to take the medicine. That would not be wise. There are some people taking statins and other drugs who have no other alternative. Those drugs all but make a natural approach impossible for these people.)

In order to understand what we mean, it's important to understand at least a little about how these Rx diabetic drugs accomplish their goal—and their side effects. Then realize that when you start down this path, you are almost certainly going to be on it for the rest of your life. That is the plan. That is why diabetes is a $35 billion per year industry—which is expected to grow to $55.3 billion annually by 2017. The bottom line is, literally, there is no profit in curing the disease. You should realize that up front.[1]

How Does the Rx Diabetic Drug "Metformin" Work?

This is a little technical, but it gives you a professional answer to the "how" of metformin. It's been in use since the 1950's, so it has a long track record of usage and research. This is one area where we really don't want just our opinions to influence you. You need to hear how the top researchers and medical practitioners see it. In this case we chose the prestigious Johns Hopkins Children's Center for the answers (Re: diabetesincontrol.com – "New Information on How Metformin Works"):

How Metformin Works

> "Not only has new research told us how metformin really works, but a new biomarker was found that can determine the optimal dose of metformin that should be used to get the best results for each patient.
>
> "Research from the Johns Hopkins Children's Center reveals that the drug most commonly used in type 2 diabetics who don't need insulin works on a much more basic level than once thought, treating persistently

elevated blood sugar—the hallmark of type 2 diabetes—by regulating the genes that control its production. Investigators say they have zeroed in on a specific segment of a protein called CBP made by the genetic switches involved in overproduction of glucose by the liver that could present new targets for drug therapy of the disease.

"In healthy people, the liver produces glucose during fasting to maintain normal levels of cell energy production. After people eat, the pancreas releases insulin, the hormone responsible for glucose absorption. Once insulin is released, the liver should turn down or turn off its glucose production, but in people with type 2 diabetes, the liver fails to sense insulin and continues to make glucose. The condition, known as insulin resistance, is caused by a glitch in the communication between the liver and pancreas.

"Metformin, introduced as frontline therapy for uncomplicated type 2 diabetes in the 1950s, up until now was believed to work by making the liver more sensitive to insulin. The Hopkins study shows, however, that metformin bypasses the stumbling block in communication and works directly in the liver cells.

"Senior investigator, Fred Wondisford, M.D. who heads the metabolism division at Hopkins Children's, tells us that, 'Rather than an interpreter of insulin-liver communication, metformin takes over as the messenger itself. Metformin actually mimics the action of CBP, the critical signaling protein involved in the communication between the liver and the pancreas that's necessary for maintaining glucose production by the liver and its suppression by insulin…'"

"Another important finding in the study: investigators have discovered a biomarker that can predict how well a person will respond to treatment with metformin and help doctors determine the optimal therapeutic dose, which can vary widely from person to person. The Hopkins team has found that in mice, metformin changes CBP in white bloods cells—just as it does in liver cells—creating a molecular marker that is easily measured via a standard blood test.

"This is the quintessence of individualized medicine: we have found an easily obtainable biomarker with great predictive power that can tell us whether and how well an individual will respond to treatment and help us determine the best dose right away instead of trying to do it by trial and error,' Wondisford says. Researchers caution that, while promising, their findings must be first replicated in humans."[2]

What are the Side Effects of Metformin?

This is the other big question and the one which obviously concerns people the most. If I take this Rx drug as prescribed by my doctor, what sort of side-effects am I likely to experience? Again, we looked to several of the experts (you can do a Web search and confirm it for yourself) and found that they all had pretty much the same list. The thing that caused us to pause and think long and hard about whether to take this medicine was just how **long** the list was!

We decided the best route was to give it to you as we found it. If you had a Top 5 "best of the best" list of medical centers and research facilities in the U.S., the **Mayo Clinic** would be on almost everyone's list. Here is their list of the drug's side-effects:

Side Effects

Drug information provided by Micromedex:

"Along with its needed effects, a medicine may cause some unwanted effects. Although not all of these side effects may occur, if they do occur, they may need medical attention. Check with your doctor if any of these side effects occur:

More common

1. Abdominal or stomach discomfort
2. cough or hoarseness
3. decreased appetite
4. diarrhea
5. fast or shallow breathing
6. fever or chills
7. general feeling of discomfort
8. lower back or side pain
9. muscle pain or cramping

10. painful or difficult urination
11. sleepiness

Less common

1. Anxiety
2. blurred vision
3. chest discomfort
4. cold sweats
5. coma
6. confusion
7. cool, pale skin
8. depression
9. difficult or labored breathing
10. dizziness
11. fast, irregular, pounding, or racing heartbeat or pulse
12. feeling of warmth
13. headache
14. increased hunger
15. increased sweating
16. nausea
17. nervousness
18. nightmares
19. redness of the face, neck, arms, and occasionally, upper chest
20. seizures
21. shakiness
22. shortness of breath
23. slurred speech
24. tightness in the chest
25. unusual tiredness or weakness

26. wheezing

Rare

1. Behavior change similar to being drunk
2. difficulty with concentrating
3. drowsiness
4. lack or loss of strength
5. restless sleep
6. unusual sleepiness

Some side effects may occur that usually do not need medical attention. These side effects may go away during treatment as your body adjusts to the medicine. Also, your health care professional may be able to tell you about ways to prevent or reduce some of these side effects. Check with your health care professional if any of the following side effects continue or are bothersome or if you have any questions about them:

More common

1. Acid or sour stomach
2. belching
3. bloated
4. excess air or gas in the stomach or intestines
5. full feeling
6. heartburn
7. indigestion
8. loss of appetite
9. metallic taste in the mouth
10. passing of gas
11. stomachache

12. stomach upset or pain
13. vomiting
14. weight loss

Less common

1. Abnormal stools
2. bad, unusual, or unpleasant (after) taste
3. change in taste
4. difficulty with moving
5. discoloration of the fingernails or toenails
6. flu-like symptoms
7. joint pain
8. rash
9. runny nose
10. sneezing
11. stuffy nose
12. swollen joints

Other side effects not listed may also occur in some patients. If you notice any other effects, check with your healthcare professional.

Call your doctor for medical advice about side effects. You may report side effects to the FDA at 1-800-FDA-1088."[3]

Maybe we are over-reacting, but that seems like a long list of potential problems to us. This motivated us to search for a possible alternative. Again, if we had no other choice and could find no other natural alternative to successfully get our blood glucose under control we would not hesitate to take this medicine.

There are literally dozens of other Rx diabetes medications on the market today—not including insulin. The ubiquitous TV ads testify to how lucrative this market is. Here is a link to the Mayo Clinic website which gives you a list of about two dozen of the most commonly prescribed Rx drugs used for the treatment of type 2 diabetes.[4]

We encourage you to check it out for yourself. At the end of the day, we were convinced that if a natural, non-Rx drug alternative existed, we wanted to find it and try it. ASAP!

Chapter 4

Understanding How to Win the Type 2 Diabetes Battle

> If we could give every individual the right amount of nourishment and exercise, not too little and not too much, we would have found the safest way to health.
>
> –Hippocrates

It is important to understand that you are now on defense in this battle. You have lost a lot of ground and your enemy is in control of it. Your soldiers (especially your pancreas) are suffering from battle fatigue. They have fought valiantly, but they are exhausted. You have to get them off the front line.

There are only two variables that *you* can control in this battle. They are your diet and how you exercise. Fortunately, they may be all you need to control and win the battle.

What Do You Do When You Are Exhausted?

That's easy—you rest, right? And that's what your pancreas needs now: relaxation, rest, and restoration. Sounds simple—and it is!

Your pancreas is not a racehorse; it's more of a plow horse.

It can run short sprints when it needs to, but that is not what it's meant to do. Like a plow horse, treat it right, give it the nourishment it needs, and it should give you many years of amazingly dependable service. What does it need? Let's deal with exercise first.

No Pain, No Gain?

I have enjoyed vigorous exercise all my life. Competitive sports have been part of my life since I was seven years old. When you are competing for excellence in just about anything, the popular maxim, "no pain, no gain," is probably true. Success has a cost.

But in this situation at least (getting control of your diabetes), that does **not** have to be true.

I guess it also depends on your definitions of *pain* and *gain*! To some folks, running the Boston Marathon would not be considered painful at all. They forget all the pain of training because of the psychological reward of finishing the race. But for me, to even walk the Boston Marathon would be agony. There would be no reward that could offset the pain. It has no appeal for me.

The reality with diabetes is that there is no alternative to exercise. It is not optional—it's essential. In other words, you can't succeed without it. Why?

Exercise *requires* your body to use its energy reserves. How does it get that energy? It gets that energy by "burning" the sugar/glucose in your bloodstream.

That is surely an oversimplification of a number of complex metabolic processes, but that's the bottom line. It first burns the glucose in the blood, then, if it needs more, it will begin using what is stored in the muscles, the fat, and finally the organs.

The reason exercise is so crucial is that it is the quickest and surest way to get excess sugar out of the bloodstream. If you can get an immediate *burning off* of sugar in the blood, this energy-*burn* will result in your blood glucose level going down, and therefore, keep it from getting "stored" in your bloodstream.

The good news is you don't have to be training for a marathon to make a real exercise impact on your blood sugar level. Moderate exercise will usually suffice. Most of us who have been diagnosed with diabetes have extra pounds we need to lose anyway—it just seems to come with the territory. So our immediate goal should be to do enough exercise to get our body to draw energy, first from the glucose in our bloodstream, then from the stored sugar (glycogen) in our fat and other organs.

How much exercise do we have to do? What kind of exercise works? The kind that eventually produces a little sweat.

You Know the Nike Admonition: *Just Do It!*

There really is no bad answer…and no pat answer. Ultimately, the key to success, as it is in so many things, is just to do it. Getting started is truly half the battle.

When I started, it was in the middle of an unusually cold winter, so my options were limited. I enjoy playing golf, and in Atlanta, we usually get a few good days (even in winter), when the weather breaks and we can play a round of golf.

When I was able to do this, I realized my blood sugar numbers came down noticeably on those days. It didn't take us long to figure out that the effect of being able to get out, walk in the sun for three to four hours (even with mild exercise), was productive in the process of getting my blood sugar under control.

But most days, I couldn't do that. So, my main exercise was limited to walking indoors. On the days when I could walk in the neighborhood, I did that. On the other days, I had to walk on the treadmill.

For the first few months, I tried to walk about two miles per day. I should admit that I hate to walk on the treadmill. I tried to walk one mile in the morning, and another mile in the late afternoon or in the evening. I tried to do it about an hour after my main meals to help work off the food. It was a bit boring, but I had no alternative. Exercise is **not** optional for a diabetic. I really did not want to be on Rx medicine the rest of my life—*so, I just did it.* **Nike** would be proud. Music, especially upbeat music, helped to keep me going. Find out what works for you.

I found the key in walking was **not** so much the *intensity* of the exercise as much as the *consistency*. I started slowly, then sped up, got to the place where I would "break a sweat" and then slowly wind down. I got to the place where I would sometimes walk on the treadmill for just 10-12 minutes at a time.

I believe it was the consistency that paid the real dividends.

Fortunately, it's summer now, so I can add swimming—which is good, because I hate to walk on the treadmill (Did I mention that!).

The point is that exercise helps to stimulate all the organ functions, yet allows the pancreas some time to rest and rejuvenate. Why? Because you're burning many of the carbs you ate before your body had to provide insulin to manage them. It's a real win-win situation for your body.

I know many people have issues that make exercise difficult, especially those of us over the age of fifty. You may have blood pressure problems or vision problems; you may have back issues, knee issues, foot or ankle issues—any number of things that make even the most basic exercise regimen a challenge. How can you deal with that?

The best suggestion I can give is this: be creative. If you have knee or back issues, find some exercise machines that will allow you to get the "cardio" you need, without putting pressure on the joints, and generating pain and inflammation.

Many believe that bicycling is one of the best exercises out there. You can go at your own pace, but you can also ramp it up any time you want. If this is too much, there are reclining bicycles where you just lie on your back and cycle. Elliptical machines are another possibility. Swimming may be one of your best options if mobility is an issue. You *can* get exercise without the stress of weight.

If these are too expensive for you to purchase (and some are quite expensive), try researching a local gym membership…or even your county recreation and parks department. Many counties have programs that offer a full range of exercise options—from exercise classes geared to specific age groups to full-fledged gyms where you can get all the exercise you want at a surprisingly low cost (these are your tax dollars at work!).

The bottom line is that to succeed in this battle, you should figure out how to get some exercise. It can start small and grow; don't despise the small beginnings! It's not where you start, it's where you end up that counts! It's a simple medical fact that your body is designed to function best when it's allowed to sweat—at least some! It's also a fact that when you allow those endorphins to be released through exercise, you just feel better.

Okay, enough on pain.

Diet is Critical

Even though it is a 4-letter word, it's really **not** a dirty word! But I know that is exactly the connotation for millions (especially those who have been on the yo-yo, up-and-down, diet-and-weight-loss treadmill—trying to lose weight by artificially stimulating the metabolism—or just starving it). It's a "dirty" word because it simply reminds them of failure—and rightfully so.

Diet is a totally different approach. It is the other key variable over which **you** have personal control in the battle with your blood sugar levels. Obviously, this makes it a huge factor.

Why? Simple. Because eating what you have been eating is most likely where the biggest changes need to take place. This is the place where you can have the biggest impact in getting control of your blood sugar problem, and allowing your body to heal itself.

Remember: Your *ultimate* **goal** is to *restore* your pancreas to a healthy state so it can process the sugar out of your bloodstream efficiently and effectively. What are the key steps to restoration?

Key Steps to Restoration of the Pancreas:

1. ***Stop the Abuse!*** What does this mean? It means eliminating the things that put your pancreas in the "sprint mode." Like what? The usual suspects. Refined sugar products, high fructose corn syrup, cokes, pastries, potato chips...you get the picture. This is Enemy #1.

2. ***Portion control.*** What does this mean? It means just what it sounds like: Anything that says "Mega" is your mortal enemy when it comes to food. It's not just **what** you eat—it's also **how much** you eat that determines your ability to succeed. *Portion control* is a huge factor in your new life as a diabetic. Why?

Part of what you must do to give your pancreas the rest it needs to be restored—is simply **not give it so much to do!** Obviously, the American diet—especially the diet offered by the fast food industry—has majored on making that virtually impossible. How? By giving us more food for less money! It's hard to turn down that "monster" deal. But the fact is this: It is turning diabetes into a national epidemic.

3. ***Balance*** is another key factor. What do we mean? When we talk about a balanced diet, we mean not only the **size** of the portions you eat, but the **variety** of the foods you eat. Your body needs not only the right size portions of food, it also needs the right balance of protein and carbohydrates and fats.

Some carbohydrates (e.g., sugar drinks, refined sugars, juice concentrates), will enter the bloodstream quickly; other *carbs* will enter more slowly. One causes what we often call a sugar spike; the other allows your body time to process the carbohydrates into energy before the system gets overloaded, and the body has to store the sugar to handle the onslaught. It is usually stored as fat.

4. ***Timing is everything.*** What does this mean? No food after 7:30pm at night.

Does that sound extreme? For those of us who have been used to having a nice bowl of ice cream (or worse) later in the evening, it might sound that way. But your body needs rest. Your pancreas needs rest. The best rest is not to make your body work. It really is that simple.

Think about this. Food is intended to supply energy to your body, right? But later in the evening, you're headed to bed. Do you really need more energy? No, you need more rest…and so does your body. Eating late puts stress on the body. How? Because you are not using up the energy you just created, and now the body has to store it. You are setting yourself up for defeat. You don't want to do this.

Here's a secret: If you want to lose weight, not eating after 7:30 p.m. is one of the best kept secrets around!

Here's another secret: If you go to bed by 9-10 p.m., you may find that you don't have the same desires for the late night snack. What's really happening is that you are already tired and looking for something that will help keep you up a little while longer. Too often the answer is to load up with sugar carbs. If you just go to bed earlier, you might find you are better off in every way. Seriously, try this and see for yourself.

You might protest that you really are hungry, and you know that the ice cream or other snack will provide at least temporary satisfaction. Your body *is* telling you something, it *does* have a need. The problem is the way you are satisfying that need. What your body is saying is that it needs fat. Fat satisfies—and fat tastes good! Fat is what makes most foods taste good.

So, is there any way to satisfy this desire in a healthy way? Yes, there is. You just have to clear away some of the confusion and misconceptions about fat. Let's try to do that now.

Chapter Five

The Truth about Fat(s)

> Did you ever see customers in health food stores? They are pale, skinny people who look half-dead. In a steak house, you see robust, ruddy people. They're dying, of course, but they look terrific!
>
> –*Bill Cosby*

The truth is, if we had a choice, most of us would much rather eat in a steakhouse than a health food restaurant. Why? It *tastes* better. Why is that? Much of what is labeled "health food" has little or no fat. Why is that? Because we have been told for at least two decades that fat is bad for you. Is that true? Yes and no!

What is the truth? The truth is that **bad** fat is bad for you. But it is also true that your brain needs fat to function properly. Am I serious? Absolutely! But—it needs **good** fat.

"Yup, our brains are made up of **60 percent fat**," says Dr. Michael Green, research psychologist at Aston University. To function optimally, our brains *need* to maintain this level of **fat.** A lower amount of fat, in fact, can lead to neurological disorders. Dieters beware! That's not a message we hear very often.[1]

It would not surprise me if researchers in the coming years discover that the modern low-fat or no-fat diet crazes of today are a primary, if not significant, factor in the development of the dementia/Alzheimer's disease. The indiscriminate goal of this type of diet may have resulted in the removal of too much good fat instead of just removing the bad fats. Fat enables all kinds of bodily functions to operate properly (especially our brain functions) and eliminating it causes all kinds of unforeseen complications.

Here's something else to consider. Does it seem strange that we have so many young kids being diagnosed with autism?

There is literally a ten-fold increase in children being diagnosed with autism in the last forty years. Remember, autism is a brain development malfunction. For the most part, these kids are perfectly healthy otherwise. Scientists are beginning to think about all kinds of possible reasons. Could it be that *cutting too much good fat* (as in excessive yo-yo dieting by the parents) could be part of the problem? We'll see in the future. (Here's a good link on autism: www.autismspeaks.org).

In the meantime, with our focus on diabetes, we need to understand how crucial the good fats are to our ability to normalize blood sugar.

While the American Diabetes Association (ADA) has softened its position on the limitations and uses of fat in recent years, the recommended diabetic's diet, in our opinion, still has a way to go. Their "unhealthy" list includes saturated fats from perennial favorites such as: chicken or turkey (with the skin), chocolate, butter, 2% milk and whole milk, cheese, etc. Of course, too much of any of these can create real problems, but with the right portions in balance, we have included them in our diets with great success.[2]

Unless you plan to live like a squirrel (surviving mostly on nuts), it can be difficult (and certainly less enjoyable) subsisting on that type of diet. Besides, if you think positive and wait five years, their advice is likely to change again.

It is always good to remember, they don't call medicine a science (even though much of it is based on science), they call it a *practice,* and for good reason! It is also wise not to forget on whom they are *practicing*. You!

Why Does *Fat* Have Such a Poor Reputation?

Let's dispel some myths—and correct some unhealthy misconceptions. The short answer is ignorance. We have been programmed to immediately relate the idea of fat to the ring of "jelly around our belly." In our culture, that is not an attractive idea.

Albert Einstein summed it up well:

> "The devil has put a penalty on all things we enjoy in life. Either we suffer in health or we suffer in soul or we get fat."

But bad dietary fat is also a *different kind* of fat. Is there no way to win in all of this?

Let's start with some simple basics...and remove some of the ignorance. Much of this is science, but it's *not* rocket science. We don't have to be able to build an engine to drive a car. We just need to be familiar enough with the parts and how they work together to get us where we want to go. And since my body is like my car, I am pretty familiar with a lot of the parts! That *personal* knowledge will be critically important information as we go through this. You know better than anyone how your body reacts.

Some Basics on *Fats*

We are not going into all the science and chemistry about fats; it is beyond the scope of this book [Editor: If you want to do research, go to the websites for American Heart Association, American Diabetes Association, or American Dietetic Association. You will find lots of information—maybe more than you want!] For our purposes, we just want to give you an overview of what we have learned.

When you go to the doctor and he reads your cholesterol results, it seems eerily similar to a police officer reading you your rights! Life as you know it may never be the same! Anyway, he tells you what the LDL, HDL, and the triglyceride levels are. What is he actually telling you? He is telling you what the levels of *fats* are in your blood. Ideally, you want low levels of LDL (low-density lipoproteins) and triglycerides and higher counts of HDL (high-density lipoproteins) fats.

Why? Are these fats really important? Can you do without them? Not if you want a quality of life you will enjoy. Again, hear the NIH (National Institutes of Health) experts:

> "Triglycerides, cholesterol and other essential fatty acids—the scientific term for **fats the body can't make on its own**—store energy, insulate us and protect our vital organs. They act as messengers, helping proteins do their jobs. They also start chemical reactions that help control growth, immune function, reproduction and other aspects of basic metabolism.[4]
>
> **The cycle of making, breaking, storing and mobilizing fats is at the core of how humans and all animals regulate their energy."**

Obviously, fats are critically important to our health. Here's the amazing thing:

> "Despite fat's importance, **no one yet understands exactly how** humans store it and call it into action." [5]

Summary: We need to grasp this. Fats are crucially important to us. Many bodily functions could not occur without them. They are the key to our body having the energy it needs, not only to get out of bed, but also to run our immune system and protect our vital organs. But "No one yet understands how…" it does it! But that doesn't stop the health-care providers from practicing on us with their latest drug ideas (especially the cholesterol-lowering statin drugs). Below is an excerpt from a Medical News Today article which highlights to us the guinea pig role we are playing in all this:

> "One of the world's most widely used drugs, statins, have been hailed by the medical community for their ability to prevent heart disease Still, the researchers who have published their findings in the journal *Diabetes* were **confused** as to why diabetes was linked to statin use.
>
> "'Recently, an increased risk of diabetes has been added to the (**FDA**) warning label for statin use,' says lead author Jonathan Schertzer, assistant professor of Biochemistry and Biomedical Sciences, and Canadian Diabetes Association Scholar.
>
> "'This was perplexing to us,' he continues, 'because **if** you are improving your metabolic profile with statins you should actually be *decreasing the incidence of diabetes with these drugs, yet, the* ***opposite*** *happened.*'"[6]

To us, that is a **very** important conclusion these medical experts are acknowledging. If statins are *causing* diabetes in many people, you have to ask, "Is the cure worse than the cause?"

This is just one more reason to try to treat diabetes without medication, if at all possible. Being forced to add one Rx drug on top of another is a prescription for disaster. Did you know that over 100,000 people die *annually* from adverse drug events? (See the bonus preview, *The Rx Drug Survival Kit* at the end of this book for more information.)

According to this team, around **13 million people** could be prescribed a statin drug at some point in their lives.

In January of 2014, the Food and Drug Administration (FDA) released a Consumer Update outlining some of the risks associated with taking statins, which included an "increased risk of raised blood sugar levels and the development of type 2 diabetes."[7]

To say that these *experts* are clueless might be a bit harsh. But they clearly do not have all the pieces of the puzzle yet (though sometimes they act like they do). We believe this gives us reasonable justification (and increased motivation) for not wanting to jump into the "pen" with the other guinea pigs—at least until we know that we have no other choice.

It's good to be cautious and see if there is not a better way—at least for you. A good doctor will agree with this statement: The best patient is a well-*educated* patient.

So, if good fats are good and bad fats are bad, what differentiates them?

Good *Fats* vs. Bad *Fats*

Dietary fats fall into two categories: good and bad. While that may sound simplistic, it is also helpful since only recently have we started to hear much about the really beneficial, indeed, the truly *essential* need for fats.

What makes *good* fats good and *bad* fats bad? Among other things, a major key is ***how it is produced.*** **Bad fats tend to be *processed.* Good fats tend to be unrefined (i.e., have very little processing).**

Under the category of ***bad fats***, is what is called *trans* fats. That is the preferred term to describe what is formally known as *"partially hydrogenated fats."* These fats became infamous because virtually all fast food restaurants used them to cook their food. Since Americans have continued to consume more and more fast foods, the impact on our diets and our health has been equally devastating. They are terrible, no other way to say it. They should, and likely will soon be outlawed.

Here's how the *American Heart Association* defines it:

> "*Trans* fats (or *trans* fatty acids) are created in an industrial process that adds hydrogen to liquid

vegetable oils to make them more solid. Another name for *trans* fats is ***partially hydrogenated oils.***

There are **nine** calories in every gram of fat, regardless of what type of fat it is. That's a lot of calories compared to carbohydrates and proteins, which contain **four** calories per gram.

Because fats are so energy-dense, consuming high levels of fat—regardless of the type—can lead to taking in too many calories. That can lead to weight gain or being overweight. Consuming high levels of saturated or trans fats can also lead to heart disease and stroke. Health experts generally recommend replacing saturated fats and trans fats with monounsaturated fats and polyunsaturated fats while still limiting the total amount of fat consumed.[8]"

Okay, let's translate this. What makes *trans* fats so bad? They are ***artificial.*** They are an *unnatural* fat that is created primarily to avoid the problem of cooking grease becoming rancid, and thus unusable. In other words, if the producer can use the cooking fat longer, it will cost less to make the food he's selling. At the end of the day, it's all about the money. Here's the NIH Medline Plus expert's comment:

"**Trans** fatty acids are manufactured fats created during a process called hydrogenation, which aims at stabilizing polyunsaturated oils to prevent them from becoming rancid and to keep them solid at room temperature. They may be particularly dangerous for the heart and may pose a risk for certain cancers.

> Hydrogenated fats are used in stick margarine, fast foods, commercial baked goods (donuts, cookies, and crackers), processed foods, and fried foods."[9]

[*Editor*: The FDA is currently considering outlawing all trans fatty acids, so this may soon be a moot point in our diets.]

Another potentially bad fat, according to the AHA, is saturated fat? What foods contain *saturated* fats?

According to the American Heart Association:

> *"**Saturated** fats occur naturally in many foods. The majority come mainly from animal sources, including meat and dairy products. Examples are fatty beef, lamb, pork, poultry with skin, beef fat (tallow), lard and cream, butter, cheese and other dairy products made from whole or reduced-fat (2 percent) milk. These foods also contain dietary cholesterol."*[10]

[*Editor*: We believe that it is the processing and homogenizing that destroys the good fats in milk and eliminates all the digestive enzymes that is causing most of the modern complaints about milk, not the milk itself.]

> *"In addition, many baked goods and fried foods can contain high levels of saturated fats. Some plant foods, such as palm oil, palm kernel oil and coconut oil, also contain primarily saturated fats, **but do <u>not</u> contain cholesterol.**"*[11]

We wonder if this doesn't come pretty close to "throwing the baby out with the bath water."

Remember, the overriding approach in most of mainstream

medicine is that to solve your cardiovascular problems, the solution is to get rid of anything that appears to raise cholesterol. Cholesterol is viewed as the key to everything. As you'll see, we don't believe this is the only viable hypothesis.

We think the culprit is more likely inflammation. Hence, we believe foods that have saturated fats (like unrefined coconut oil), enjoyed in moderation, are perfectly healthy and can even be very helpful in getting blood sugar under control. We will present the evidence we have found, but you have to decide this issue for yourself.

But We Need *Fats*! Right?

No, we need *good* fats. One thing we said above needs to be remembered. No matter what fat you're talking about, even the good ones will have twice as many calories (which we need for energy) than protein or carbohydrates.

This is where *portion control* and *balance* are critical. You need to include *good* fats in your cooking and diet, but they also need to be in balance. If you miss this, you may be eating a healthy diet, but you may also gain weight. This is almost always a battle for those with diabetes. We will give you examples in the chapter on *Meal Plans and Recipes*, so you will know what we really mean by portions and balance.

So, if *saturated* fats (like the ones we've been describing) are bad for us, what kinds of fats do we include?

[Note: Remember, we do *not* agree that all saturated fats are bad, so when you see us including fats that we think are quite healthy for us, you will know why.]

But according to the experts, we also need the *unsaturated* fats (which includes both the mono- and poly-unsaturated fats). Where do we find them?

For this, the virgins aren't good enough, you will want the *extra virgin* oils.

What's the difference? It's mostly about the processing. The less processing you have, the better the quality of fats (in this case and in most cases, we are talking about oils).

We are not going through all the potential candidates, but we are highlighting a few that will serve us well. Let's start with oils that most everyone agrees should be on the list, and which are very economical and widely available.

Olive Oil and Other Favorite Oils

Obviously, the medical experts would like our choices of oils to be either a monounsaturated or polyunsaturated oil. Basically, we agree with this. But trying to remember all the technical distinctions can get tedious. And above all, we want this book to be of *practical* use to you—and in real life, we know that people will only use (and continue to use) things that they like.

In general, we would suggest that a good, healthy oil comes from health-giving plants, seeds, or fruits. It needs to be as close to organic as possible, and should be cold-pressed, extra virgin, and have a fresh smell—not rancid.

Your oils should be kept in dark bottles if possible and away from heat, except for cooking, to help maintain freshness.

(Remember: Unrefined oils have no preservatives and will not stay fresh forever. Rancid oils will usually taste quite bitter. They may even make you sick, so store oils properly and use them frequently.)

There are some oils which are probably best avoided altogether. The primary reason is that they are usually highly processed oils (which enables them to last longer without spoiling). Why is excess processing bad?

Processed oils are usually refined in a way that is *not* particularly healthy. Some use chemical extraction, others use heat. If heat is used in any way, as we all know, it tends to destroy. Usually it destroys flavor as well as health benefits. Besides, the best stuff is usually not much more expensive, so it's really worth it. Many of these oils have been linked to serious diseases, including cancer and heart diseases. Just a partial list would include: soybean oil, canola oil, corn oil, rapeseed oil, etc.

That's a long list of "not so good." Are there any really healthy alternatives? Absolutely! Olive oil, for one, meets all our needs.

Olive oil: a superior heart-healthy oil, has become the poster-child for healthy oils. You can use it raw as a dipping oil, or for salad dressings, etc., not to speak of being on virtually everyone's *best-of-the-best list* these days when it comes to a cooking oil.

You can find all kinds of cold-pressed extra virgin specialty olive oils online (it just depends on how much you want to spend). If you want a nice grocery store option, try the *California Olive Ranch* extra virgin olive oil/first cold-press. It's reasonably priced, tastes very good, and has no unpleasant aftertaste.

Another great undiscovered oil is **avocado oil.** It has many of the same characteristics as olive oil. If you have never tried it, you might find that it's another great addition to your cooking choices.

Having said that, there are some very healthy, good-tasting oils that don't cook well. **Walnut oil** is one of them.; it adds an exquisite flavor when added to salads, fruits and fresh cooked vegetables and many sauces., but it doesn't cook well and can become bitter with heat; it's best used at room temperature.

Likewise, there are some oils which have a great deal of nutritional health value (like fish oils and seed oils) which are great to use as supplements, but should also be avoided for cooking purposes.

An "Under-the-Radar" Diabetic's Jewel

Just a quick note on another favorite oil of ours—***extra virgin* coconut oil.** This has been an overlooked, hidden gem. We'll address this oil in more detail in Chapter Seven where we discuss "(Almost) Magical Preservatives."

Suffice it to say, the use and effectiveness of extra virgin coconut oil has been terribly under-appreciated in years past, but that is changing. Once you realize its benefits you will likely never be without it again. We sure won't.

Coconut oil can be bought unrefined and in about as natural a state as you could want—make sure you buy the *real* thing!

The more refined (i.e., processed) it is, the lower the quality you are buying. For an excellent overview article on cooking oils, check out the one by Authority Nutrition on healthy oils. [12]

There's another really great cooking oil, but it only has friends in the culinary camps: **Butter!** Is it really so bad? Honestly, we don't think so.

Chapter 6

Butter, Cholesterol, and Inflammation: An Inconvenient Truth?

Be careful about reading health books,
you may die of a misprint.

–Mark Twain

IF you believe the mantra of mainstream medicine (i.e., that most cardiovascular diseases are caused by cholesterol build-up in the arteries), you may want to skip this chapter. We think the answer lies in a completely different cause and this chapter contains some of the reasons why. We believe that inflammation, *not* cholesterol, is the real culprit. And if cholesterol is not the real problem, then cutting out the benefits of butter (both culinary and otherwise) is a mistake. Butter may even help to *reduce* inflammation.

We know that butter has gotten a bad "rap" over the past few years. Why? It is what is called a *saturated* fat, which means it is "bad" (i.e., it raises your bad cholesterol), which in turn makes you a more likely candidate for cardiovascular disease. We believe this is totally true when describing margarine, but we are not so convinced about butter.

The facts are that supposedly over 75% of the cholesterol in your arteries is laid down by your mid-twenties. Is that true?

If so, then you would want to control or slow down the damage that is potentially being done to the **last 25%**. Let's assume this is true (maybe it is, but maybe not). The real question is this: Is trying to reduce cholesterol by *statin* drugs really solving the underlying problem? Also, we think it is important to ask whether the side-effects (which can be horrendous) are worth the cost (both physically and financially).

Statins and Cholesterol

Remember, how do *statins* work? They work by causing your liver to produce less cholesterol. This doesn't sound too bad...until you start considering what the "collateral damage" to that monkeying with the liver functions might be causing! It's just a fact of life, when the liver shuts down, so do you. This is Medicine 101.

There is strong evidence for an *alternative* belief that it is ***not*** cholesterol that is causing this wave of cardiovascular disease, it is *inflammation.*

Don't take our word for it, hear an undisputed authority:

> "'Although it is not proven that inflammation **causes** cardiovascular disease, inflammation is **common** for heart disease and stroke patients and is thought to be a sign or atherogenic response. It's important to know what inflammation is and what it can do to your heart,' added Deepak Bhatt, M.D. (President of the American Heart Association).

"'Exactly how inflammation plays a role in heart attack and stroke remains a topic of ongoing research.'

"'Cholesterol-lowering medications called statins **appear** to reduce arterial inflammation, but whether that's from cholesterol reduction **or** something else is being debated,' Bhatt said. 'He added that clinical trials are ongoing to see if other medications might lower inflammation in arteries and reduce the risk of heart attack and stroke. More information on the role of inflammation should be available in the next few years.'"[1]

Okay, let's unpack this a little bit. Anyone who has watched TV has seen some of the many commercials touting the need to *get your cholesterol down,* and of course, there's a *statin* drug to help you do that. There are at least **ten** Rx drugs available to do that...and they are hugely profitable for the drug companies. That, it strikes me, might be a motive for them to take a long, long time to see if those *"other medications might lower inflammation in arteries and reduce the risk of heart attack and stroke."* Seriously?

What the doctor appears to be saying is simply this: Cholesterol might *not* be the real problem; inflammation might be the culprit. We think the *statins* are helping to reduce the cholesterol counts, but we don't know if the real reason is actually because they are reducing the inflammation! Might be. We'll see in a few years.

Maybe I am being a bit cynical here, but it sounds to me like what they could be saying is this:

"When the profits on the statin drugs start declining, we'll likely start promoting and selling inflammation-reducing drugs." That, of course, is just my opinion.

With the incredibly scary list of the *statin* drugs' side-effects (they can literally take up one to two pages or more of an ad in a magazine!), I would like to consider my alternative options for some anti-inflammatory treatments ***now***, that is, if I can find them.

Fortunately, you can. And some of them are in foods you can eat! And, there are other *natural* options.

[Editor's note: Why are we including this information on inflammation in a diabetic diet treatment book? Good question. *It just so happens that the same approach to reducing inflammation (for heart disease) also helps get blood sugar under control.* Do you think that's just a coincidence? We do not. So, as you read about reducing inflammation *naturally*, we believe you are likely looking at one of the best ways to control blood sugar as well. Below is a quote from another expert, Dr. Russell Greenfield, which represents a true paradigm shift from traditional medical thinking about the source of disease and the impact diets may have on their treatment.]

Why Anti-Inflammatory Diets?

The simple answer is that for many people they work. Just like there are dozens of different Rx drugs to get your cholesterol down, there are also many variations on the anti-inflammatory diet theme. Some target different types of inflammation (colon vs. allergies vs. high blood pressure, etc.).

The common theme is that they all recognize that many components of the modern diet (which is heavily sweetened) lead to constant, and eventually, chronic inflammation.

The conclusion is that a body that is under constant attack from inflammation simply cannot effectively fight off disease. When it finally succumbs, the scene can get very ugly and painful. The bottom line is, as assistant professor of medicine at UNC Chapel Hill, Dr. Russell Greenfield concludes, ***"It is very clear that inflammation plays a role much more than we thought with respect to certain maladies."*** [2]

These doctors make it clear that the traditional mindset in mainstream medicine operates on the basic premise that if a disease is identified as an "itis" then its source is likely to be related to inflammation in the body. Clearly, diseases like arthr*itis* and appendic*itis* would historically fall into this category, but now it's looking more and more like cancer, high blood pressure, and heart disease may also, at least in part, be caused by inflammation.

Dr. Greenfield's conclusion is a stunning admission that will likely lead to alternative treatments that do not involve or depend on prescription drugs. Maybe Hippocrates was right after all, eating right and exercising **is** the safest way to health. Imagine that!

What kind of diet promotes this ***anti***-inflammatory response in the body? Again, there are a variety of opinions, but there are common denominators among them all.

Anti-Inflammatory Diets: What Do You Eat?

An exact description of the anti-inflammatory diet varies; it just depends who you ask. In general, the anti-inflammatory diet is "probably very close to the Mediterranean diet," says Doctor Christopher Cannon, MD, associate professor of medicine at Harvard Medical School and a cardiologist at Brigham and Women's Hospital, Boston. He co-authored *The Complete Idiot's Guide to The Anti-Inflammation Diet*[3], which includes recipes for anti-inflammatory eating and information on vitamins.

Where Is the Proof That Reducing Inflammation Works?

Can a diet really affect disease-causing **inflammation** in the body?

Proponents say it can, but they acknowledge that to have an impact on the paradigm change needed to dislodge the current "lower the cholesterol with statin drugs" mindset, the anti-inflammatory diet needs to be studied more extensively. Unequivocal clinical proof that it actually reduces disease such as heart problems will be needed. In the meantime, practical and anecdotal testimonies are all around us. Even the experts acknowledge it.

"But a related diet, the **Mediterranean diet, has been and is** associated with improved cardiac outcomes," Cannon says.[4]

Greenfield agrees. "There is **ample evidence [of disease risk reduction]** on the Asian-style diet and the Mediterranean-style diet," he says.

"When you take a look at the components [of those diets], they could easily be called anti-inflammatory diets."[2]

What is he saying?

Let's put it in terms we all understand, namely, *"A rose by any other name is still a rose."* The components of the Mediterranean and Asian diets tend to include foods that reduce inflammation. All we are doing now is focusing in on that fact and pairing it with the realization that inflammation (rather than cholesterol) may be at the center of much of our modern diabetic and cardiovascular disease problems.

And remember, one of the NIH doctors we quoted earlier said he was **not** exactly sure how *statins* reduced our cholesterol…that they might be working because they are reducing inflammation!

All we are saying is this: **If** that is truly a possibility, wouldn't it be even better if we could find a natural way to reduce inflammation and accomplish the same goal without all those terrible side effects??? We think the answer is pretty obvious.

What Makes Up the Inflammation-Reducing Diet?

Again, Harvard Medical School professor, Dr. Christopher Cannon, co-author of *The Complete Idiot's Guide to The Anti-Inflammation Diet*[3], gives this general outline.

Specifics vary from diet to diet, but in general, anti-inflammatory diets suggest:

- Eat plenty of fruits and vegetables. Minimize saturated and *trans*- fats.

- Eat a good source of omega-3 fatty acids, such as fish or fish oil supplements and walnuts.
- Watch your intake of refined carbohydrates such as pasta and white rice.
- Eat plenty of whole grains such as brown rice and bulgur wheat. (Editor: Consider quinoa also.)
- Eat lean protein sources such as chicken; cut back on red meat and full-fat dairy foods. (Editor: Cut back, not cut out.)
- Avoid refined foods and processed foods.
- Spice it up. Ginger, curry, and other spices can have an anti-inflammatory effect.

As one example of a day's worth of anti-inflammatory eating, Cannon suggests a breakfast of toasted steel-cut oatmeal with berries, yogurt, or other topping, and coffee or green tea. Lunch could be tuna salad on 7-grain bread and a smoothie with seasonal fruits. For a snack, try an ounce of dark chocolate and about four walnuts. Dinner could be spaghetti with turkey meat sauce, spinach salad with oranges and walnuts, and apple cranberry pie made *without* butter. (*Ed.* We might argue with this last point!)

“The (anti-inflammatory) diets don't promise weight loss, but weight reduction does often occur. And that makes sense, given the makeup of the diet,” says Greenfield.[2]

Why does it make sense?

Because when you start eliminating things like partially hydrogenated oils, highly processed carbs (i.e., store-bought breads, cakes and anything with refined sugars or high fructose corn syrup)—and adding healthier proteins (like fish); eating more fruits and vegetables, etc.—"odds are that people are going to lose at least a little bit of weight." Sounds an awful lot like some common sense is beginning to seep into the primary health-care provider thinking here.

It wouldn't be the first time mainstream medicine changed direction on the "best way" to do something once they got more information. Sadly too often, profits have more to do with the "flow of information" than most of us realize. So, who has the most incentive to maintain the status quo? Remember, you are responsible for you. It's been well-said, ***"If you are not looking out for you, you can be sure no one else is."***

Chapter 7

Superior Supplements for Controlling Blood Sugar

(PART ONE)

> I eat organic, I take supplements as determined by lab work, I sleep eight hours nightly, I use organic cosmetics and green household cleaners, and I avoid toxins as best I can.
>
> —Suzanne Somers

It would be wonderful if we could get all our nutritional needs met from the foods we eat—and once that was possible. It's no accident that we are called "the breadbasket of the world." Sadly, the quality of what is produced is not what it once was. The once notorious abundance of natural minerals in our soils is now missing. Maybe one day everything will be set right again, but until then, the reality is, we will need to supplement what we eat with critically important nutrients in which we tend to be deficient. Like what?

Let's remember what our main problem is. Our glucose (i.e., our stored blood sugar) is not metabolizing efficiently. We are not processing the glucose so it can be used for energy. Therefore, what we need to do is accomplish two things:

First, we should give our bodies supplements to help it process our foods (and the blood sugar it creates) more effectively;

Second, we need to *slow down* the demand on the whole metabolic process as much as we can so the body can process the food without being overloaded.

Remember, the pancreas is in a debilitated state right now, and it needs time to "rehab." Too much stress too soon will only cause more harm and make it more difficult (and take longer) to reach the goal. We found that the right supplements can help relieve some of that stress. Here is what we discovered.

[Note: Earlier we told you we would give you some recommendations for places where you can get the best deals on products we have used. We list some below. However, for over-all supplement needs, one of the best online sources we have found is *Swanson Vitamins*. Prices and service are as good as you could want—and let them know how you found them.]

Before we go through the list of specific supplements which we have used and found beneficial in addressing blood sugar issues, we need to start by making sure you are building on a solid, dietary foundation. Like what? I would suggest that there are some key elements which are especially important to someone dealing with blood sugar issues—a potent, high-quality daily multi-vitamin, chromium, magnesium, and an excellent source of B-vitamins.

Why Are B-Vitamins So Important?

B-vitamins are your *stress* vitamins. They undergird your immune system more than any other vitamin. You need to make sure you are getting an ample supply of your B-vitamins.

The list of reasons is endless, but the bottom line is that we all live under debilitating stress. Stress is the silent killer in our lifestyle and culture today. You can't avoid it, so you had best protect yourself. The B-vitamins do this.

There are two ways to approach this—pills or powder. Most people opt for a pill. That is fine; just make sure the list of B-vitamins is long and potent. We use an excellent B-vitamin supplement marketed by *Young Living Essential Oils*. The product is called *Super B*. My wife has difficulty taking many B supplements as they can be hard on the stomach causing her to feel nauseated. *Super B* is easy on the stomach and doesn't cause her any adverse effects. If you are looking for an excellent Vitamin B supplement, consider *Super B*. You can order it at: www.youngliving.org/rebekahbrazier.

There is also a powder alternative often described as *nutritional yeast*. I have used *YeastPlus* product for over 30 years for two reasons. The primary one is that *nutritional yeast* is reputed to be the most natural and complete source of your B-vitamins—and I wanted to make sure I was getting them all. This brand also includes almost all the amino acids and (as I mentioned earlier), it also has a special Chromium supplement (called GTF Chromium) which helps me metabolize sugar.

Why was this important? Honestly, thirty years ago I had no idea. I assume now the Lord was just looking out for me. Below I have included some of the comments from one of many studies that now recognize the need for chromium in the type 2 diabetic's diet.

Unless you are a chemist, you might not understand it all. I don't either. But what I do get is that there are medical doctors who are *not* normally favorably disposed to the idea of the use of supplements, yet the results were strong enough that they had to admit that there seemed to be a positive impact for type 2 diabetics who added GTF chromium to their regimen. FYI: You can also buy GTF Chromium as a stand-alone supplement.

Here is what the diabetes experts said:

> "Interest regarding chromium administration in patients with diabetes was kindled by the observation in the 1970s that it truly was an essential nutrient required for normal carbohydrate metabolism. A patient receiving total parenteral nutrition (TPN) developed severe signs of diabetes, including weight loss and hyperglycemia that was refractory to increasing insulin dosing (3). Based on previous animal studies and preliminary human studies, the patient was given supplemental chromium.
>
> "In the following 2 weeks, signs and symptoms of diabetes were ameliorated, with markedly improved glycemic status and greatly reduced insulin requirements (exogenous insulin requirements decreased from 45 units/day to none). Other studies (4, 5) of the beneficial effects of chromium in patients receiving TPN have also been documented in the scientific literature. Chromium is now routinely added to TPN solutions (5).
>
> "The results of these studies strongly implicated chromium as a critical cofactor in the action of insulin

> (6, 7). Whereas chromium replacement in deficiency states is well established, the role of chromium supplementation to enhance glucose metabolism in subjects is controversial and serves as the basis for this review." [1]

Regardless of what you choose, just make sure you are starting with a high quality multi-vitamin and/or a supplement with a good quality B complex like *Super-B,* if needed. Understanding the need for that solid foundation, let's look at two of the special supplements we used to get our blood sugar under control. We start with chromium because as we researched it, we found it to be one of the most richly documented supplements in the treatment of type 2 diabetes. It was so essential we quickly added more to our daily regimen.

Chromium

For whatever reason, diabetics seem to have a deficiency in both chromium (and magnesium as well). Thirty years ago, someone talked me into getting a hair analysis. I thought it was silly at the time, but the one thing I do remember is that it came back showing I had—you guessed it—a chromium deficiency, at 30! Of course, I had no idea what to do about it, but here is where the Lord was looking out for me in my ignorance.

It was at that time that I was introduced to Twinlab's *YeastPlus* product which had a specially added supplement called "GTF Chromium". The GTF stood for Glucose Tolerance Factor. In other words, it was targeting a blood sugar problem I didn't even know I had. It probably helped to stave off my diabetes for many years. It didn't have enough in it to fix it completely, but I am sure it helped to delay the problems I eventually developed.

I originally began taking the product to address stress problems in my twenties. Your B-vitamins supply get depleted when you're under a lot of stress, regardless of your age. One way or the other, you need to meet the deficiency that the stresses of our modern daily life is creating on all of us.

FYI: We believe stress is also a major factor in developing diabetes. It leads to bad eating habits and it also leads to organ stress overload. It also appears to lead to the inflammation that may result in diabetes.

Remember, our real goal was *not* just to get the blood sugar under control, it was also to address the core problem which was causing the body *not* to be able to process the blood sugar efficiently.

The fact that the supplement was addressing a huge chromium deficiency was totally lost on me at the time, but now I am beginning to appreciate its value.

The experts vary in their recommendations on just how much chromium you need to get your type 2 diabetes and insulin resistance under control. Dr. Mark Hyman suggests in his blog that you take 200–600 mcg of chromium polynicotinate per day.[2] Aware that I previously had a chromium deficiency, I decided to go a little stronger.

For the first 3 months, I took one Swanson 1000 mcg chromium product called *Chromax 1000* in the morning, then at dinner, I took two 200 mcg capsules of Swanson *Albion Chelated Chromium.*

Since the doctors cited above concluded that "chromium is very important for proper sugar metabolism," I felt it was important—and I experienced no negative side effects that I could identify.

You should start with the doctor-recommended amounts and then add more if needed.

You can find all kinds of information on chromium on the internet. Much of it is from highly reputable, mainstream medical sources. Here are some fundamental facts you will discover in your research:

Chromium. Chromium is an essential trace element. It is also a metal. Ultimately the chrome plating on your automobile is sourced from chromium. Obviously, you don't want to "chrome plate" your organs and arteries, so you only need minute traces. Yet, it is still an essential element for some bodily processes. That is why it is called an *essential trace element*; only very small amounts of chromium are necessary for human health.

For people who have been diagnosed with diseases requiring them to be on steroids or statins, developing diabetes is often unavoidable, especially if they were "borderline" or in the pre-diabetic stage to begin with (as some 80 million Americans are).

Chromium was originally discovered in the 18th century, but it was the mid-1960s before its true value as an essential trace element was identified. Modern applications for chromium include weight management and decreasing body fat. Some believe that chromium can increase energy and improve athletic performance. The bottom line is that it is an essential element in achieving and maintaining good health.

How Does Chromium Work?

Chromium appears to help keep blood sugar levels normal by improving the way our bodies use insulin. If used as directed, there normally appears to be no adverse side effects. However, if you are already taking diabetic medications or have liver disease, WebMD offers the following warning:

> "Chromium might *lower* blood sugar levels too much if taken along with diabetes medications. If you have diabetes, use chromium products cautiously and monitor blood glucose levels closely. Dose adjustments to diabetes medications might be necessary.
>
> "There are *three* reports of liver damage in patients who took chromium picolinate. Don't take chromium supplements, if you already have liver disease."[4]

[*Editor: Considering that it is likely that millions of people have taken chromium supplements, three was not a number that concerned me.* ***But if I had liver disease or were already taking medication for diabetes, I would pay very close attention to how I reacted to chromium.***

More than one prescription drug has been known to cause liver damage, so make sure to pay attention to what happens to yours!]

If you want some eye-opening insight on the damage that Rx drugs are having on this country, check out this book at Amazon.com: ***The Rx Drug Survival Information Kit.***

Most people are totally unaware that Rx drugs are a leading cause of death in America, with over *100,000 deaths each year resulting from adverse drug reactions!* You do not have to be a victim of this plague. A simple test can usually give the doctor the right information to get you the right drug at the right dosage. One size does **not** fit all when it comes to Rx drugs!

Magnesium

Magnesium is another remarkably beneficial supplement. It is a mineral and it has tremendous ability to help relax your muscles. Most folks don't realize it, but when a person has a heart attack, often the first thing the hospital should do is put you on a "magnesium drip." Why? To help relax the heart muscle which has cramped.

It also greatly aids in glucose metabolism. Nationally recognized diabetes expert, Dr. Mark Hyman, recommends around 400-600 mg per day.[5] You may experience a loosening of your bowels if you get too much. If you have a tendency toward constipation that may be good news. If not, you may have to scale down and take less. Your body will usually tell you what it needs; learn to listen to it!

Unlike chromium (which is a metal), magnesium is a mineral. It makes up a large part of the essential mineral needs of the body, especially the bones and muscles. It helps relax the muscles—it helps strengthen the bones. Experts estimate that the body contains around 25 grams of magnesium. It is involved in over 300 chemical reactions in body processes.

Ideally, people should get sufficient magnesium directly from the foods they eat. If magnesium levels are too low, a supplement may be necessary. Low levels are noticeably more prevalent in women than in men, and more so among African-Americans than Caucasians, as well as among the elderly of all races.

You can identify foods that are good sources of magnesium by looking for foods with high *fiber* content. Green vegetables tend to be good sources: leafy greens, seaweed, dried beans, grains, and most seeds and nuts. For those who love chocolate, this is a great excuse to indulge (a little bit anyway). Chocolate is a good source of magnesium, especially the darker varieties.

If you have ever lived in a place with "hard water" (like the folks living in Florida!), you know what we are talking about. Hard water has a high mineral content. Magnesium is one of the minerals that produces the effect. Drinking this water can supply *some* of your magnesium needs if the taste is not destroyed by other sanitizing processes. When I lived there, the water in Florida was virtually undrinkable, which is why the bottled water industry flourished there before it did in so many other places.

The variety of uses for magnesium almost seems endless. It is used for all types of cardiovascular disease treatments, from irregular heartbeat to high blood pressure. Many believe it can be a key element in the natural treatment of ADHD issues, and others, not surprisingly, find it effective in dealing with RLS (restless leg syndrome).

How Does Magnesium Work?

Magnesium performs many functions in the body. We need it especially for the growth and maintenance of our bones and muscles. Without magnesium our nerves and muscles will not function properly. In the stomach, magnesium helps to neutralize stomach acid and move stools through the intestine. Ever heard of "Milk of Magnesia?"

Magnesium is one of the most underrated minerals in our diet. The number of people who are deficient and don't know it are probably legion. What ultimately opened our eyes to its value was when we discovered that one of the standard operating procedures at many hospitals is to put heart attack victims on a magnesium drip as soon as possible.

Why do they do this? Magnesium relaxes the muscles (and our hearts are arguably our most important muscle!).

Deciding on your dosage is an interesting challenge. The daily recommendations provided by the experts vary widely. We take at least one 400 mg capsule daily. Whichever brand you choose, you may want to start with their recommended dosage. It is easy to determine when you get too much—you'll experience diarrhea. In that case, just lower the dosage until you determine your tolerance level. Most health professionals want you to add calcium whenever you supplement with magnesium. Here are some links to help you.

See – drhyman.com – 5 Steps to Reversing Type 2 Diabetes and Insulin Resistance
Also – care.diabetesjournals.org – content/28/51175.full

Chapter 8

Superior Supplements for Controlling Blood Sugar

(Part Two)

L-Arginine and Niacinamide

According to the NIH (National Institute of Health), "*Proteins* are large, complex molecules that play many critical roles in the body. They do most of the work in the cells and are required for the structure, function, and regulation of the body's tissues and organs."[1] Why is this important?

Proteins are made up of amino acids. *L-arginine* is an amino acid. These amino acids are what allow the "worker bee" proteins to do their jobs effectively. Without them the human body simply is not able to work effectively, if at all.

L-arginine can be obtained from the foods we eat or it can be created in a laboratory. Natural sources include red meat, dairy, fish and poultry products—foods we would normally think of as sources of protein.

L-arginine is also used as a form of medicine. Its applications are well-known and often very effective—sometimes stunningly effective!

It is widely known for its blood vessel relaxing or expanding capabilities. Consequently it is used for conditions such as high blood pressure, coronary heart disease, and congestive heart failure. Some have used it to relieve RLS (Restless Leg Syndrome). Others have combined it with ibuprofen and found relief from migraines.

The bottom line in all these applications and the resulting effectiveness is that it improves blood flow—and most of these ailments have as their root problem some form of obstructed blood flow. Anecdotal evidence suggests some have found success or improvement in dealing with both erectile dysfunction and senile dementia.

Do you struggle with cold hands or feet? Many diabetics do. You might want to try an l-arginine supplement and see if increasing the blood flow in your body helps. The biblical declaration that "the life is in the blood" is not an idle one; it can be the difference between a high quality of life and a miserable one.

How Does L-Arginine Work?

In layman's terms, L-arginine helps arteries to expand and thereby improves blood flow. "L-arginine is converted in the body into a chemical called nitric oxide. Nitric oxide causes blood vessels to open wider for improved blood flow. L-arginine also stimulates the release of growth hormone, insulin, and other substances in the body."[2] That is why it may help diabetics.

The doctors at the **Mayo Clinic** concur (www.mayoclinic.org):

> "**Arginine** becomes nitric oxide (a blood vessel-widening agent called a vasodilator) in the body. Early evidence suggests that arginine may help treat medical conditions that improve with increased vasodilation. These conditions include chest pain, atherosclerosis (clogged arteries), heart disease, heart failure, erectile dysfunction, peripheral vascular disease, and headaches from blood vessel swelling)."

The problem is that our arteries tend to harden, constrict and become clogged as we age and indulge in poor eating habits. When the hardening or constriction becomes severe enough, a heart attack may occur. Arginine helps those hardened arteries to relax to allow increased blood flow. The more our blood flows freely throughout our body, the more energy and healing we can experience. Of course, the opposite is also true...which is why poor circulation can be hazardous to your health. This is critical for diabetics.

The research on this is very solid. Here is another example:

Pharmaceutical Research

In new experiments, researchers from the University of Copenhagen working in collaboration with a research group at the University of Cincinnati, USA, "*demonstrated that the amino acid arginine improves glucose metabolism significantly* in both lean (insulin-sensitive) and obese (insulin-resistant) mice."[3]

Why is this important?

These experiments appear to show that the amino acid *arginine*—found in a wide variety of foods such as salmon, eggs, and nuts—greatly improves the body's ability to metabolize glucose (blood sugar).

Arginine stimulates a hormone linked to the treatment of type 2 diabetes, and *works just as well as several established drugs on the market.* The research findings have been published in the scientific journal *Endocrinology*.

Why is this important? More than 371 million people worldwide suffer from diabetes, of whom 90% are affected by *lifestyle-related* type 2 diabetes! In other words, if you make some lifestyle changes, you can have a major impact on your diabetes, even avoiding ever having to go on Rx medicine.[4]

L-Arginine, Heart Disease...and a Doctor's Shame

We found one doctor's experience very compelling. He had been working, as so many doctors do, to get his patients' A1c hemoglobin numbers down to a normal level. And without question, there are numerous medicines available to do this, so he was successful. But he says, he was "ashamed." ***Why? Because while he was getting the blood sugar numbers down, he ended up sending one-third (240 in one year!) of his patients to the cardiologist so they could be treated for heart disease!! Why?***

It is because some of the more popular drug treatments for diabetes end up causing the heart to work harder to make up for the diabetes treatment. It was a win-lose situation. He was in need of serious help. He found it in L-arginine.

Now, instead of sending hundreds of patients the next year to the heart doctor, he sent one. That's not a misprint. What was the secret of his success? He found that arginine relaxed the arteries, improved blood flow, and reduced the severity of atherosclerosis.

Since 1993, he has treated over 7000 patients without a single heart attack or stroke. The key appears to be that the arginine is converted to nitric oxide which allows arteries to relax, blood flow to increase, and blood pressure to be lowered. His proprietary formula uses 5000 mg per day.[5]

Niacinimide is somewhat similar to arginine in that it helps to promote circulation of the blood in the arteries. It is one of the few natural supplements often prescribed for diabetics by medical doctors. It is used as a dietary supplement for those who are in the pre-diabetes stage to help increase the metabolism of blood sugar. It's part of the B-3 vitamin family. While giving many of the same benefits as niacin, it does not cause the often uncomfortable (but harmless) niacin flush. The normal dose is about 500 mg per day. I often take both.

Alpha Lipoic Acid

If you take the time to do the research, you will find that alpha lipoic acid (ALA) is designated as an *antioxidant.* There is a lot of talk today in nutritional literature about the value of antioxidants because they fight "free radicals." Unless you are already steeped in the sometimes mysterious vocabulary of nutritional descriptions, this doesn't tell you much, so let's try to put it in laymen's terms.

What are *antioxidants*? And why is it important that they "fight free radicals?" Why do we care?

When our bodies break down food into its various nutritional components so that the circulatory system can transfer it to our organs in the form of energy, not all of it is used. You could think of it in this way…

When a builder is building a house, he buys more materials than he actually needs because he knows there will be some "waste" in the building process. There is no way to avoid it.

Inside our bodies, this waste is called "free radicals." Just like in the house-building process, if you don't clean away the excess waste, it eventually gets in the way of your ability to finish building the house.

In your body, this process is called *oxidation*. This may not be the best scientific metaphor, but think of it like rust. Rust is the corrosive excess that forms when metal is oxidized, that is, exposed to oxygen in a moist environment for an extended period. Alpha lipoic acid helps to break down the corrosion so the excess can be removed, allowing nutrients to again be transported through the body, allowing it to function normally.

Alpha-lipoic acid is sometimes prescribed as a natural alternative for symptoms of diabetic neuropathy (i.e., nerve-related pain, burning, numbness in the legs and arms. German doctors are known for using high doses of alpha-lipoic acid in the treatment of these types of diabetic symptoms.

According to WebMD, "alpha-lipoic acid is also used to treat eye-related disorders…damage to the retina, cataracts, glaucoma, and an eye disease called Wilson's disease."[6]

How Does Alpha Lipoic Acid Work?

The function of alpha lipoic acid in the body is targeted to prevent the cell damage that will occur if the "free radicals" are allowed to accumulate in the body. ALA also helps to break down the *carbs* we eat so they can be converted into energy for other organs in the body.

In diabetics, ALA seems to help fight off neuropathic disease which can be extremely debilitating.

A typical recommended dosage is 300-600 mg.

Gymnema Sylvestre and Cinnamon

On virtually every natural health provider's list of blood sugar lowering supplements you will find *gymnema sylvestre*. We had never heard of it (still have trouble pronouncing it!) and we have used natural supplements for many years.

Gymnema evidently has a long history of use in India's Ayurvedic medicine. The leaves are used to make medicine. The Hindi name, *gurmar*, means "destroyer of sugar."

How Does This "Sugar-Destroyer" Work?

According to WebMD,

> "Gymnema leaves contains substances that decrease the absorption of sugar from the intestine. Gymnema may also increase the amount of insulin in the body and increase the growth of cells in the pancreas, which is the place in the body where insulin is made."[7]

The typical dosage seems to be around 300 mg per day. Some people find that gymnema sylvestre helps their weight-loss efforts. The reason seems to be that it helps decrease the absorption of blood sugar from the intestine, hence less excess glucose being stored as fat in the body.

This is clearly an added bonus for those with type 2 diabetes, since their insulin resistance often makes it more difficult to lose weight.

Cinnamon is often bundled with Gymnema (which makes sense since cinnamon is a staple of Indian cooking. It's such a commonly used spice, can it really help lower blood sugar? There is so much anecdotal testimony to this effect that many medical experts have been forced to ask the same question.

Does Cinnamon Help Diabetes?

Doctors at the Mayo Clinic, while not endorsing it, do allow that there may be benefits to including it in your diet. Dr. Regina Castro reviewed one study published in 2009 which found "that a 500 mg capsule of cinnamon taken twice a day for 90 days improved hemoglobin A1C levels—a reflection of average blood sugar level for the past two to three months—in people with poorly controlled type 2 diabetes (hemoglobin A1C levels greater than 7 percent)." So, while not declaring it a solution, it may be helpful in a regimen that seeks to control blood sugar levels.

As we all know, Cinnamon is a spice. It comes in two main varieties—Ceylon cinnamon and cassia cinnamon. Cassia cinnamon is the kind most Americans use for baking and cooking. It's also the variety most researchers have used when they've studied cinnamon and diabetes.

Multiple small studies have demonstrated what clearly appears to be *improved* (i.e., lowered) blood sugar levels associated with cinnamon intake. How does it do that?

By decreasing insulin *resistance*. How does it do that?

In people with type 2 diabetes, the sugar-lowering hormone *insulin* does **not** work as well. This leads to unacceptably higher blood sugar levels.

WebMD highlights the conflict which pits experts on both sides of the issue. "In one study, volunteers ate from 1 to 6 grams of cinnamon for 40 days. One gram of ground cinnamon is about half a teaspoon. Researchers found that cinnamon *reduced cholesterol* by about 18% and *blood sugar* levels by 24%. In other studies, cinnamon did ***not*** decrease blood sugar or cholesterol levels."[8] You have to decide. Personally, I couldn't see any downside; besides, I like the taste of cinnamon in my coffee!

Does Cinnamon Interact With Other Herbs or Drugs?

We found this warning on the WebMD site and couldn't resist including it. You need to pay attention to its warning, but you have to appreciate the irony in it…

Because cinnamon may lower blood sugar levels, exercise caution when combining it with other supplements that lower sugar levels. The same holds true with diabetes medications. If you and your doctor decide cinnamon is right for you, pay close attention to your blood sugar levels. Let your doctor know if your blood sugar levels *fall too low*" (www.WebMD.com).[9]

I love it when I see warnings like that! If I am trying to get my blood sugar under control *naturally*, I will be thrilled to see that kind of result! After all, we've already mastered the skill of getting it too high!

My doctor congratulated me and told me to keep doing whatever I am doing. Your doctor probably will do the same, so by all means, tell him if it's getting too low!

I can't tell you why cinnamon seems to work sometimes, but not others. But there is an enormous amount of anecdotal information saying that it has real impact—certainly enough to convince me to include it in my daily regimen. I like "easy," so my solution has been to put about a half teaspoon on top of my coffee grounds in the morning before I start the drip process. Everyone who tastes it thinks it's wonderful—like some gourmet blend. If you do not have an easy way to use it regularly like this, there are gymnema supplements that you can buy which often include cinnamon. [See: www.swansonvitamins.com]

[**Note**: If you are taking ***statin*** drugs, check with your doctor if you think you would like to add cinnamon to your vitamin regimen. It apparently **may** cause an adverse drug reaction in some people. ADR's are never good…and can be deadly!]

Salmon Oil and EFA's

EFAs are Essential Fatty Acids. In other words, they are fats. As we talked about earlier, fats have a bad name among many people. But it is not healthy fat that makes you fat, it is *bad* fats that make you fat and unhealthy.

The truth is, fat is brain food—at least good fats are. Dr. Mark

Hyman gives an excellent description of good fats:

> "Fat is one of the body's most basic building blocks. The average person is between 15 and 30 percent fat! Of all of the types of fats in our diets, the body only REALLY needs two—omega-3 and omega-6.
>
> "What is an *omega* fat? The omega-3 and omega-6 numbers refer to where the hydrogen atom joins the fat molecule. Remember, the name is just basic chemistry lingo. What is important is to understand the impact of different fats on the body.
>
> "The higher-quality the fat, the better your body will function. That's because the body uses the fat you eat to build cell walls. You have more than 100 trillion cells in your body, and every single one of them needs high-quality fat."[10]

Salmon oil is one of the best sources of EFAs. The normal dosage is about 1000 mg per day. The benefits of EFAs are virtually endless, they are true essentials. You can see more at his blog here.[11]

Another excellent source of EFAs is *sardines*. I know, I know, the first reaction is usually "phfew—the smell is awful!" There is no denying that it can be quite strong; we felt the same way.

However, we did find a brand of high-quality Pacific sardines that were lightly smoked and packed in extra virgin olive oil. Having them just lightly smoked seemed to help greatly! They were excellent and the smell was quite tolerable (though maybe I just told myself, "Get used to it; you need these!").

I ate them on crackers 4-5 times per week for lunch the first couple of months. They gave my body some greatly needed EFAs and, I believe, really accelerated the whole process of getting my blood sugar under control.

If you do any research on them, you will often find them listed as a "superfood." They are a high-protein, low-carb food and loaded with EFAs. You really need to try them; it's one of the finest *diabetic* foods you will ever find. The brand we like best is from Wild Planet. The best price we found was, believe it or not, at Costco, not a health food store! It ended up costing less than $2 per tin—almost half the cost of many others.

If you are looking for more information on Omega-3-6-9 oils, here is a link to a nice site with a simple breakdown of what is what and what contains what. There is no question but that these oils are essential to heart health and proper blood sugar metabolism. Just make sure the oils you choose are undamaged, i.e., cold-pressed and minimally processed.[12]

Chapter 9

Probiotics, Enzymes, and Kefir

Many of you may be scratching your head at this last one. **Kefir**. What is kefir?

We'll get to that. Let's start with *probiotics*. What are probiotics? The experts at the American Gastroenterology Association give a definitive medical description:

> "*Probiotics* are living microscopic organisms, or microorganisms, that scientific research has shown to benefit your health. Most often they are bacteria, but they may also be other organisms such as yeasts. In some cases they are similar, or the same as the "good" bacteria already in your body, particularly those in your gut."[1]

These good bacteria are part of the trillions of microorganisms that inhabit our bodies. This community of microorganisms is called the *microbiota*. Some microbiota organisms can cause disease. However, others are necessary for good health and digestion. This is where probiotics come in.

The most common probiotic bacteria come from two groups, *Lactobacillus* or *Bifida bacterium*, although it is important to remember that many other types of bacteria are also classified as probiotics. Each group of bacteria has different species and each species has different strains. This is important to remember because different strains have different benefits for different parts of your body.

For example, *Lactobacillus casei* Shirota has been shown to support the immune system and to help food move through the gut, but *Lactobacillus bulgaricus* may help relieve symptoms of lactose intolerance, a condition in which people cannot digest the lactose found in most milk and dairy products. In general, not all probiotics are the same, and they don't all work the same way. For more general information on probiotics check out the American Gastroenterology website[2]

In Layman's Terms

Okay…in layman's terms, *probiotics* are good bacteria in the "gut," but they can't efficiently do what they need to do without enzymes. What are *enzymes*? According to Healio.com (a physician-targeted website for health specialists):

> "An enzyme is a biological molecule that serves as a catalyst for chemical reactions. Enzymes reduce the amount of energy necessary to carry out the reaction, thereby allowing it to occur at an increased rate, often

> at rates millions of times faster than comparable reactions that are un-catalyzed.
>
> "Enzymes often serve in the digestive systems of living organisms. Amylase and protease are enzymes that help break down large molecules—including starches or proteins—into smaller molecules. The smaller molecules may then be absorbed by the intestines. Starch molecules are turned into maltose or glucose."[3]

What are they saying? In vastly oversimplified terms, probiotics enable us to digest our food and convert it into energy. Enzymes are the catalysts that jumpstart and accelerate the process by breaking down the food into molecules that can be digested and converted into the things our body needs to operate.

As an example, as we get older it is sometimes more difficult to digest and metabolize a large protein-rich meal, e.g., a steak. I have experienced this many times. So I will often include a capsule of HCL (hydrochloric acid) with my meal. It is an enzyme which helps break down the protein so my gut can metabolize it.

Why Is This Important, Anyway?

Glad you asked. It has been well-said that "life and death begin in the colon." How you process, digest and metabolize your food (and eliminate what is not needed) will in great measure determine the quality of life you enjoy. In other words, you may not feel sick, but do you feel well? Do you have the energetic, healthy feeling that you think you should be experiencing?

If not, this could be a major reason. There's a reason why (according to NIH statistics) over 60 million Americans suffer from chronic constipation! [4]

The seriousness of this situation is reflected in the statistics. Some 80% of Americans report experiencing constipation, about 30% claim chronic constipation. Then you have the other side of the ledger where you have people with chronic diarrhea, usually in the form of Crohn's disease, Irritable Bowel Syndrome (IBS), and Irritable Bowel Disease (IBD). The International Foundation for Functional Gastro-Intestinal Disorders (www.aboutibs.org) states that between 25 and 45 million Americans suffer from some form of these disorders. If you add these up, somewhere around 50% of the folks in this country have "gut" problems—and they don't feel well!

Probiotics, enzymes and kefir can help this problem. What is kefir? Here's from the folks at the *Chuckling Goat* in the UK:

> "**Kefir** (pronounced ke-feer) from either the Arabic "keyf" (joy and pleasure) or the Turkic "kopur" (milk) is a fermented drink originating with shepherds of the North Caucasus region. Kefir is a natural probiotic drink, similar to, but stronger than live yogurt.
>
> "**How is it different to yogurt?** Both kefir and yogurt are cultured milk products…they contain different types of beneficial bacteria. Yogurt contains short-lived beneficial bacteria that provide food for the friendly bacteria that reside in the gut.
>
> "It's a 'one-shot deal'—only aiding digestion while the

yogurt is actually **in** your system, so you need to keep re-introducing it to see any benefit.

"But kefir contains live active, growing living cultures of very strong strains of normal flora; these will actually **permanently** repopulate your digestive tract with good bacteria, powerful enough to overtake harmful organisms —*a feat that yogurt can't match!* [Editor: This is one reason why antibiotics are often so destructive; they can't tell the "good guys" from the "bad guys," so they wipe out all the good bacteria in the gut when they attack the "bad guys!" So, if you ever have to take an antibiotic, start taking kefir immediately and start re-populating your gut bacteria. This is especially important for young children.]

"Kefir's active yeast and bacteria provide more nutritive value than yogurt by helping to digest the foods that you eat and by keeping the colon environment clean and healthy. Because the curd size of kefir is smaller than yogurt, it is also easier to digest, which makes it a particularly excellent, nutritious food for babies, the elderly and people experiencing chronic fatigue and digestive disorders."[5]

You can read more from the folks at the links below. The bottom line is that kefir is another one of those "superfoods" that you should seriously consider adding to your diet on a regular basis. The good news is that you can find it in lots of places (even in grocery stores),—just look for it in the refrigerated health food section.

Here's a bonus: Do you struggle with *acid reflux*? Indigestion? I know the experience of waking up in the middle of the night with that burning sensation in the back of my throat. It's no fun.

If this happens to you, try a couple of ounces of kefir. It solves my problem every time. I am not a fan of plain yogurt or plain kefir (though my wife is); fortunately the Lifeway brand that we buy has several flavored versions. It is only about $3.99 a quart (at the time of this writing) and seems to last forever for me. It is delicious. Yes, it does have a little sugar to sweeten it, but it's a price I am willing to pay to get the long-term benefits of kefir, and it takes care of the acid reflux problem, for me anyway. My wife on the other hand has gone full-tilt into growing and culturing her own kefir grains. FYI: the real stuff is about ten times more potent that the product you buy in the store.

Resource links that might give additional insights:

http://diabetesdietdialogue.wordpress.com/2009/06/12/diabetics-need-probiotics/

http://imperfectlynatural.com/kefir-the-wonder-probiotic-drink/

If you want to learn how to make your own, here is another source:

http://www.culturesforhealth.com/Kefir/

Chapter 10

(Almost) Magical Preservatives

> Older people should **not** eat health food, they need all the preservatives they can get.
>
> –Robert Orben

As we progressed through this diabetic recovery journey (especially the arduous process of assessing the abundance of information, both accurate and inaccurate, then attempting to distil it into useful form for ourselves—and others), we uncovered several things that we believe are so valuable we will never again be without them.

Anti-aging products are big business today. The stated goal is to enable you to live longer. Few would argue with that desire. However, though it is rarely articulated, the underlying assumption is that we all want to live longer **and** enjoy a good quality of life. The sad fact is this: with all the government interference, it is getting harder and harder to die, let alone enjoy a good quality of life! Too many of us are living longer, but enduring a very poor quality of life health-wise.

This is something that should be addressed and planned for as early as possible, if we are to enjoy a healthy lifestyle in our later years—and we are not talking about long-term care insurance.

LTC insurance surely has its place, but wouldn't it be better to be proactive in providing you and your family with better long-term health! That's our goal.

There are four food supplements which we believe are almost magical in their ability to give you the greatest chance of creating a high quality of life and health over the long term. They can help everyone, but they may be especially helpful to the diabetic, and by extension, to those with heart disease. Here they are: raw (not processed) apple cider vinegar (ACV), extra virgin coconut oil, organic whey protein (from grass-fed cows), and black cumin seed oil.

There are endless testimonies that multitudes of users have given on these products. The "experts" call this anecdotal (i.e., non-scientifically verified) evidence. Does this mean these testimonies are not credible? No. It just means they could not (or have not tried to) reproduce the results in a lab. We think there are good reasons to include these foods in your diet regimen—and we will try to share them. We also urge you to take special note of the distinguishing characteristics that we point out. Ignoring these can keep you from experiencing the enormous benefit of these products. Here is just one example.

You can buy apple cider vinegar in lots of places. But if you don't get ACV which still has "the mother," you have probably wasted your money. We will explain why, and again, we'll try to give you some suggestions where you can get many of these high quality products at the best prices.

Magical Preservative #1

Raw Apple Cider Vinegar (with the *mother*)

The anecdotes for apple cider vinegar are so ubiquitous even WebMD had to comment on it!

> "You probably have a bottle of apple cider vinegar in your pantry right now. It's a tasty addition to homemade pickles, marinades, and salad dressing, but is it also good for you?
>
> "As a folk remedy, apple cider vinegar has been credited with curing everything from the flu to warts. Many of its supposed benefits are unproven, but some experts think that adding a little of this sour liquid to your life may have some health benefits."[1]

Clearly, the WebMD folks don't give it a ringing endorsement, but some medical professionals are a lot more convinced.[1]

Apple Cider Vinegar and Blood Sugar

While apple cider vinegar probably won't make you skinny, it does appear to help with diabetes and blood sugar control.

After studying apple cider vinegar for more than 10 years, Carol Johnston, PhD, director of Arizona State University's nutritional program, believes the effects of apple cider vinegar on blood sugar are similar to other *prescription* medications.

"Apple cider vinegar's anti-glycemic effect is very well documented," Johnston says.

She explains that the vinegar blocks some of the digestion of starch. "It doesn't block the starch 100%, but it definitely prevents some of that starch from being digested and raising your blood sugar," Johnston says.[2]

But not every expert feels as confident about apple cider vinegar's power. Here's the other side of the argument.

"Trying to use vinegar to treat diabetes is like trying to bail out a flooded basement with a teaspoon," says Michael Dansinger, MD, director of Tufts University's diabetes lifestyle coaching program.

He advises patients to focus instead on their overall diets—a strategy backed by a lot more research, he says.

If you have gastroparesis, a common problem with diabetes that slows stomach emptying, be careful. Early research shows apple cider vinegar may make this problem worse.

"I'm concerned that drinking vinegar, even diluted in water, increases acid in your system, which puts a strain on your kidneys and bones," Dansinger says.

But Dr. Oz has a different take on this. He believes it *stimulates* the digestive juices. He also believes it can be a helpful solution for everything from dandruff to sore throats.[3] See the footnote for a blog entry from Swanson Vitamins's nutritional experts listing thirty uses for raw ACV—and about as many ways to incorporate it into your daily diet.[4]

As noted in the footnote above, one of the best and most reliable brands of organic ACV is produced by the Bragg's company.

The legend of Paul Bragg goes back to the 1920's when he is credited with being the "Father" of the natural health food movement in America. He opened the first health food store and later, the first health food restaurant in the U.S. But by far his most famous and lasting legacy is the raw and unfiltered ACV product which bears his name.

It's easy to see why Bragg's has such a high reputation when you read the ingredients and certifications on their flagship product. It is USDA certified as organic; so you don't have to be concerned with pesticide poisoning. Here is the way the product label reads:

> "Certified Bragg Organic Raw Apple Cider Vinegar is unfiltered, unheated, unpasteurized and 5% acidity. Contains the amazing **Mother of Vinegar** which occurs naturally as strand-like enzymes of connected protein molecules.
>
> **Information:**
>
> "Bragg Organic Raw Apple Cider Vinegar is made from delicious, healthy, organically grown apples. Processed and bottled in accordance with USDA guidelines, it is Certified Organic by Organic Certifiers and Oregon Tilth; and is Kosher Certified. Bragg Organic Raw Apple Cider Vinegar is full of zesty natural goodness. Non-GMO Certified. It's a wholesome way to add delicious flavor to salads, veggies, most foods, and even sprinkle over popcorn.

> "Apple Cider Vinegar has been highly regarded throughout history. In 400 B.C. the great Hippocrates, Father of Medicine, used it for its amazing health qualities. **No refrigeration required."**

That's the label. The thing I want you to pay particular attention to (and which should be on the label, or the website, of whatever brand of ACV you buy) is the phrase "Mother of Vinegar." This is what distinguishes vinegar which is alive from the stuff that has no nutritional value.

What is "the mother"? Any vinegar that is clear and has no "mother" (the strand-like substance in the bottom of the bottle) has little, if any nutritional value. Period. The "mother" is only obtainable in raw, unfiltered, and unpasteurized apple cider vinegar.

Bragg's says:

> "Make sure you use raw, organic vinegar, never dead, distilled vinegar because the natural enzymes, minerals, and nutrients are destroyed in the distilling process. Natural raw ACV should be pungent, with a rich, brownish color and a visible "mother." Drinking apple cider vinegar daily, and eating a largely fresh, organic, vegetarian diet, along with following a simple fitness program, will change your life so dramatically you will never go back to your old ways."

We're not big believers in the vegetarian approach (though lots of really good folks are); otherwise, to us, this sounds like good advice for diabetics.

Our Testimony: From the second week into this research and recovery odyssey, we began to create our own dietary regimen for getting my diabetes under control; obviously, raw ACV was one of the first products we included. We chose to get it in a product called *Yoder's Good Health Recipe (more on that below).* We could not ignore all the testimonies to its benefits. In the end, we determined "it certainly can't hurt to include it." We are SO glad we did.

Specifically, for the first three months, we included it at each meal, three times a day. We normally drank one-half ounce (1 tablespoon) at each meal. At first we didn't even dilute it, though eventually we did. It is pretty tart, and diluting it does not seem to affect its benefits.

[Point to Note: Most purveyors of ACV strongly encourage you to dilute it (usually in 5-8 ounces of water or juice), and you may want to even use a straw to drink it. Why? It's an acid, which can be hard on your teeth. This will help keep it off your teeth as much as possible. If it's still too tart for you, try adding a teaspoon of organic honey (or maple syrup, blackstrap molasses or stevia) to sweeten it.]

Another thing to note: if you use Bragg's AVC, it is *very* economical. We can buy a 32 ounce bottle from Swanson Vitamins for under $5.00. That is very helpful to the budget.

Full Disclosure: "Yoder's Good Health Recipe"

As mentioned above, just a few weeks into this odyssey, we came across a particular concoction of apple cider vinegar that appealed to us. My wife had already done a great deal of research on herbs and such that were believed to help get blood sugar under control. One day she was in a local farmer's market and came across a product called **Yoder's Good Health Recipe**. The basic ingredient was apple cider vinegar, but it also included fourteen *other* herbs and spices, some of which we had already identified as aids in our quest—things like ginseng, cinnamon, fenugreek, etc. Their raw ACV drink (with the *mother*) was also mixed with organic apple juice and a few other things that made it taste a bit better than just raw apple cider (though it was still pretty tart and needed to be diluted).

We decided that we would try it and for the next three months it became the daily ACV staple of our diet. We have never regretted this decision.

Having said that, the one downside is that it is a bit pricey—about $18-$24 for a 25-ounce bottle. But since we only used one-half ounce at a meal, we felt it was worth it.

Bragg's ACV is a lot more economical, but if we hadn't started with the Yoder's, we might never have known how valuable raw ACV really is. If you can afford it, you might want to get Yoder's 4-bottle option and try it for a month—at least for now. This option gives you a 20% discount (at the time of this writing). Either way you go (Bragg's or Yoder's), raw apple cider vinegar is, in our view, an essential pillar in a diabetic recovery regimen. For more info, here are the web addresses of these two companies: (www.yodersstore.com) and (www.bragg.com).

Magical Preservative #2: Extra Virgin Coconut Oil

We mentioned this a little earlier, but it bears repeating—this is also an essential ingredient in your fight to control type2 diabetes! Extra virgin coconut oil (EVCO) is what the biochemists call an MCT (a medium-chain triglyceride).

That is a technical term for a type of fatty acid. Medium chain triglycerides, or MCTs, have a shorter chemical composition compared to most other fats and oils. They also are lower in calories than long chain fatty acids. MCTs (like coconut oil) are quickly absorbed by the body and used as energy, whereas long-chain fatty acids are stored as fat by the body.

The product researchers at Swanson Vitamins give us this analysis of coconut oil and why it is so valuable compared to other fats.

> "For years coconut oil got a bad rap because of its nature as a saturated fat. But the more researchers learn, the more they're reversing their original conclusion that all saturated fats are damaging to health. (The fats to completely avoid are trans-fatty acids and hydrogenated and partially-hydrogenated fats.)
>
> "Saturated fats come in two forms—those that are comprised of medium-chain triglycerides (MCTs) and those that are made up of long-chain triglycerides (LCTs). Coconut oil is an MCT, and these forms of fat are not stored in our cells like other forms; rather, they are easily digested and sent to the liver where they are immediately converted into energy. [Editor: Who doesn't need more of that?]
>
> "Additionally, coconut oil (used in moderation) does not clog the arteries nor does it raise LDL cholesterol levels. On the other hand, LCTs like those found in butter and

other animal-source saturated fats are stored in the cells. Animal fats also contain cholesterol and can actually raise LDL cholesterol levels, so they should be consumed very sparingly.

"Coconut oil is ideal for cooking (even at higher temperatures), baking, or eating straight out of the jar. Unlike polyunsaturated fats that quickly turn rancid, coconut oil is highly stable. *Even after a year of no refrigeration, it shows zero evidence of rancidity.*

"This quality automatically moves coconut oil to a highly preferred status because rancid or spoiled fats wreak havoc on our health, creating a free radical nightmare inside the body."[5]

If you know anything about oils, you know that rancidity is a **big** problem. The bottom line is that having a little coconut oil with most of your meals will help slow the sugar uptake into your blood-stream. Why?

Because it is quickly and easily converted into energy, instead of being stored as fat! Besides, the good stuff really tastes good.

Where to buy it inexpensively. We have tried the products from a number of online health food stores (Swanson, Vita-Cost, etc.), and they all have quality products and decent prices. For example, this week Swanson is selling its 16 ounce Organic EV coconut oil for $8.49; its 54 ounce bottle is $21.89. **Their sales change constantly**, so always check.

[**Note**: It is critically important that you get *extra virgin* coconut oil, preferably organic. Make sure what you buy is **not** hydrogenated! It should be extra virgin, and even better, cold-pressed oil. One is very bad for your heart, the other is very good for it.]

(FYI: The real stuff congeals (solidifies) below about 76 degrees and melts into a liquid above that temperature. It is best stored in a cool, dry place. True EVCO is whitish in color.)

We found a brand produced by Carrington Farms that is super quality and the 54 ounce bottle costs about $17.00-$18.00.

If you can't find it locally, you can try an online option called *Boxed*. It's an online grocery store that is competing with Amazon pantry and some others for your grocery purchases. For first time buyers (at least for now), they are offering a 15% discount plus free shipping. It is definitely worth checking out.

What if I don't care for the coconut flavor? This wasn't a problem for me because I love the flavor. But not everyone does. We hear that Spectrum Naturals has an organic, *refined* oil in which the aroma is not noticeable. You might want to try that. The bottom line is that extra virgin coconut oil belongs in your daily regimen.

Magical Preservative #3: Organic Whey Protein

WebMD is right when it declares:

> "High-protein, low-carbohydrate diets are the hottest thing since sliced flank steak, and every food marketer in the known universe appears to want a piece of the protein pie.
>
> Body builders are snatching, grabbing, and gulping

> down protein shakes. Dieters are gobbling down protein bars (and shunning pasta) in hopes of quick weight loss."[11]

Most of us first heard about protein drinks because body builders made it one of the key elements of success in building a body which has more muscle than fat! What they don't tell you (or at least you have to read the fine print to find out) is if you don't plan to do lots of exercise, too much protein can turn to sugar, then stored as fat—so the whole plan can backfire on you!

That's not to say, it's not good for you (after all, we've included it in the "Magical" section). But you can waste a lot of time and money if you don't get the right stuff. There are an awful lot of whey protein products that could almost qualify as junk food.

Protein is essential, there's no question about that. It is the building block for almost everything in your body, from muscles to organs.

As WebMD says:

> "It's easy to understand the excitement. Protein is an important component of every cell in the body. Hair and nails are mostly made of protein. Your body uses protein to build and repair tissues. You also use protein to make enzymes, hormones, and other body chemicals.
>
> "Protein is an important building block of bones, muscles, cartilage, skin, and blood."[12]

That just about covers everything. The body stores fat, but it does not store protein, so you have to supply it regularly, one way or another.

Why Is *Whey* Protein So Good?

Because it contains all the essential amino acids. It is a complete protein, and it can build virtually anything. In addition, it carries the highest quality rating of any protein.

What Is the Source of Whey Protein?

It is a by-product of the cheese-making process. It was once considered basically worthless; at best it was used as animal feed. But nutritional research eventually realized its value to humans and the rest as they say, is history. Use any search engine to find out all you could ever want to know.

If it comes from cheese then it comes from cows; it is a dairy product derivative. If at all possible, choose a whey product that does not come from cows that are being fed or shot up with all kinds of chemicals, antibiotics, and hormones. Eventually, you get what they get, so you need to be careful. Fortunately, there are good sources of grass-fed, hormone-free whey protein available.

Dr. Joseph Mercola, one of the most popular, online good nutrition gurus, has summarized the keys to look for in a quality whey protein. He lists about nine different things that are important:

1. **All-natural, pasture-fed cows' whey, *NOT* pesticide-treated, grain-fed cows' whey**

   Compared to grain-fed cows, pasture-fed cows produce whey that:

   - Is nutritionally superior to grain fed

- Contains an impressive amino acid and immuno-supportive nutrient profile
- Is rich in healthy fats—lipoic acid and CLA (conjugated linoleic acid)

2. **GMO (Genetically Modified Organism)-*free* Whey**

   Choose whey made without GMOs.

3. **Cold processed, *NOT* heat processed**

   Most whey is heat processed which:

   - Makes the whey acidic and nutritionally deficient
   - Damages the immuno-supportive micro-nutrients and amino acids
   - Makes whey inadequate for consumption

   Cold processed whey protects the nutrients in their natural state.

4. **Acid-*free* processing, *NOT* Acid / Ion Exchange Processing**

   Acid/Ion Exchange Processing is cheaper than acid-free processing, but it denatures the amino acid profiles by using acids and chemicals to separate the whey from the fats.

5. **Whey protein concentrate, *NOT* protein isolates**

   Protein isolates are proteins stripped away from their nutritional co-factors. There are three problems with that.

   - All isolates are exposed to acid processing.
   - Your body cannot assimilate proteins in isolated form.

- Due to over-processing, isolates are deficient in key amino acids and nutritional co-factors.

You must make sure you get whey protein concentrate instead of protein isolates, which are an inferior product.

When you remove fat, you actually remove components of its immunological properties, such as phospholipids, phosphatidylserine, and cortisol. Additionally, all of the igG immunoglobulins, which are an excellent source of glutamine and cysteine, are also bound to the fat globule. Fat provides not only calories; most foods rich in healthful fat—including nuts and seeds like almonds and chia—are carriers of antioxidants, such as vitamin E and phytosterols.

Therefore, you're clearly left with an inferior whey protein if you take the fat out. So don't settle for anything less than whey protein concentrate.

6. **Sweetened naturally, *NOT* artificially, and low carb**

   Most whey products are artificially sweetened making them useless if you have sugar sensitivities, or just don't want to put artificial sweeteners or flavors into your body.

   Your whey should be low glycemic, low carb and should not contain any artificial sweeteners, sugar alcohol, glycerin, fructose, sugar, or gluten.

7. **Maximum biological value, *NOT* compromised or damaged**

Most whey proteins provide *some* benefit. But due to the ingredients, the source of the whey, the concentration of beneficial nutrients, or the type of processing, many whey products simply don't deliver what they promise.

You want whey that's guaranteed to retain its maximum biological value—one with all the key amino acids, co-factors and beneficial micro-nutrients present and intact rather than compromised or damaged, and not missing any amino acids or essential nutrients.

8. **Easy to Digest, *NOT* Causing Digestive Stress**

Many whey products contain long-chain fatty acids, which are hard to digest and require bile acids to absorb.

You want a whey protein powder with medium-chain triglycerides (MCT). These are easily absorbed, digested quickly, and utilized as energy without causing digestive stress.

Ideally, you want a product in which the MCT comes from the best source of all—coconut oil.

9. **Free from Toxic Heavy Metals or at Such Low Levels *NOT* to be a Health Risk**

Many protein powders both whey and non-whey could contain dangerous levels of heavy metals like mercury, lead, cadmium, and arsenic.

A *Consumer Reports'* evaluation showed that some leading brands of protein powders exceeded United States Pharmacopoeia's (USP) recommended safety limits for certain heavy metals.

> You want to avoid these products at all costs because any high concentration of heavy metals taken over time could lead to serious health consequences."[13]

Okay, that is Mercola's recommendations, and of course, he markets a high quality product. It's a little pricey for me (at about $25-$30 for a 16 ounce can), but the quality should be excellent. We receive no financial benefit for mentioning this. See the footnote above if you want to try it.

After all our research, we were just as happy with the Swanson brand whey protein which was from grain-fed, certified rBGH-free cows and produced excellent whey protein. You can get it in a vanilla, chocolate, or strawberry flavor, and it's about half the price of the Mercola brand. You might want to try one of each and see what works best for you.

Both of these are high quality products. The Swanson grass-fed certified whey can be found at *www.swansonvitamins.com.*

Proteins are one of the absolutely essential building blocks of life. *Whey protein is especially good for diabetics.* As pointed out above, it is easily digested and has all the amino acids the body needs to build, repair, and heal itself. It is an almost perfect food. It is low-carb, high-protein, and best of all, there is no sugar issue because there is no sugar! This is one product you should seriously consider including in your blood sugar conqueror's regimen.

Magical Preservative #4: Black Seed Oil/Black Cumin Seed Oil

This is probably the best kept secret of all—at least in the western world. The truth is, black seed oil has been used for thousands of years in the Middle East, and was even found in the tomb of a famous Egyptian king. It has even been said that this oil is the remedy for all diseases except death.[13]

No doubt, that is a strong endorsement, but is there any basis in fact for it? Actually, there is a stunningly large amount of research documenting its usage.

What Is Black Seed/Black Cumin Seed Oil?

For those who have never used them as resources, it sometimes comes as a surprise to find out that there is a vast wealth of medical/biomedical research available—usually for free, drawn from research done all over the world, and on virtually every subject related to health. These are your tax dollars at work. Part of them go to fund the NIH (National Institutes of Health) and many related sources (e.g., PubMed, PubMed Central). It is a treasure trove of information, ***if*** you have the time and desire to use it. Obviously, most of us don't have the time or the need. But when you want to know what is going on in the biotech/biomedical world, this is a great place to start. And there is all kinds of research focused on Black Seed Oil.

The official botanical name is Nigella Sativa, hence black seed which is commonly used as a flavoring or spice. We know it has been in use for over 3,000 years because it was found in the tomb of King Tutankhamun, better known as King Tut of Egyptian fame. [14]

Historically, black seed has been used to treat ailments such as headache, toothache, and even intestinal worms.[15]

Today, its primary medicinal constituent is the extracted black seed oil. Applications of black cumin seed oil are focused on conditions which are primarily viewed as inflammation-related (inflamed/irritable bowels, colitis, etc.).

It is also believed to be effective as an aid in treating upper respiratory conditions including asthma, allergies, bronchitis, emphysema, etc.[16]

One of the more dramatic applications was the incorporation of black cumin seed oil in combination with several other natural components to lessen the side effects of a cancer chemotherapy drug (cisplatin). This drug is used to treat a dozen different kinds of cancer, including bladder, colon/rectal, and breast cancers. Its effects were especially hard on children and this concoction was apparently of great help in reducing the debilitating side effects of the treatment on these children.[17]

Some people apply black seed oil directly to the skin to reduce inflammation and joint pain, most notably from arthritic type conditions.

How Does Black Cumin Seed Oil Work?

WebMD gives a rather generic answer to this one:

> "There is some scientific evidence to suggest that black seed might help boost the immune system, fight cancer,

> prevent pregnancy, and lessen allergic reactions by acting as an antihistamine, but there isn't enough information in humans yet."[18]

In other words, "...We really don't know."[18]

As referenced earlier, we first heard about it being used as part of a University of Minnesota research study where cold-pressed seed oils were used to try to lessen the effects of chemotherapy (especially in children).

Again, the key seems to be its ability to reduce inflammation, boost antioxidants, and thereby boost the immune system.

Here's one summary of the potential benefits—it is a PubMed abstract of a study done at the Medical University of South Carolina. For those who don't know, *PubMed* is a subsidiary of the National Institutes of Health—in other words, this is Federal Government-recognized research on black cumin seed oil:

> "A larger number of medicinal plants and their purified constituents have been shown [to have] beneficial therapeutic potentials. Seeds of Nigella sativa (official name of black cumin seed oil), a dicotyledon of the Ranunculaceae family, have been employed for thousands of years as a spice and food preservative.
>
> "The oil and seed constituents, in particular thymoquinine (TQ), have shown potential medicinal properties in traditional medicine.
>
> "In view of the recent literature, this article lists and

discusses different immunomodulatory and immunotherapeutic potentials for the crude oil of N. sativa seeds and its active ingredients. The published findings provide clear evidence that both the oil and its active ingredients, in particular TQ, possess reproducible anti-oxidant effects through enhancing the oxidant scavenger system, which as a consequence lead to antitoxic effects induced by several insults.

"The oil and TQ have shown also potent anti-inflammatory effects on several inflammation-based models including experimental encephalomyelitis, colitis, peritonitis, oedama, and arthritis through suppression of the inflammatory mediators prostaglandins and leukotrienes. The oil and certain active ingredients showed beneficial immunomodulatory properties, augmenting the T cell- and natural killer cell-mediated immune responses.

"Most importantly, both the oil and its active ingredients expressed anti-microbial and anti-tumor properties toward different microbes and cancers.

"Coupling these beneficial effects with its use in folk medicine, N. sativa seed is a promising source for active ingredients that would be with potential therapeutic modalities in different clinical settings.

"The efficacy of the active ingredients, however, should be measured by the nature of the disease. **Given their potent immunomodulatory effects, further studies are urgently required** to explore bystander effects of TQ on

> the professional antigen presenting cells, including macrophages and dendritic cells, as well as its modulatory effects upon Th1-mediated and Th2-mediated inflammatory immune diseases. Ultimately, results emerging from such studies will substantially improve the immunotherapeutic application of TQ in clinical settings."[19]

Obviously, even if you can't understand all that is said, what is clear is that these researchers were impressed with the potency and the potential of black cumin seeds, particularly the cold-pressed oil. That is the important point.

There are literally *hundreds* of studies showing not just a mild effect, but in some cases, as much effect as chemotherapy on some types of cancers. If this type of information interests you and you want to do more research, do a Web search on PubMed..., you can search forever!

Some believe that if you take black seed oil *with honey (raw), the benefit is increased even more.*

Sources and Disclaimers

Full Disclaimer: Black Cumin Seed oil does *not* taste good, period. But whatever your source for this oil, make sure it is pure and unfiltered, cold pressed, and solvent free. Our favorite black cumin seed oil is made by Sweet Sunnah.[19]

Mix the black seed oil with honey and/or anything else you think tastes good. This oil is not cheap, but it does last a long time. We find that a teaspoon a day takes care of most of our ailments (e.g., it has almost replaced my need of ibuprofen for pain issues in my lower back).

If you prefer not to have to deal with the taste at all, Swanson Vitamins sells a good quality option in capsules for both the **seed** and the **oil** forms (I cannot taste it at all). To find it, just search *www.swansonvitamins.com* for **black cumin seed**.

That is the last of the "magical supplements" we use.

Now here's the daily regimen of those supplements that we promised you.

Chapter 11

Daily Regimen of Dietary Supplements

Here is a summary list of daily supplements and the amounts we used to get my blood sugar under control.*

Morning:

- 1 tablespoon Twinlab Nutritional Yeast (or a high quality daily supplement like Young Living *Super B*)
- 1 capsule Chromax (Chromium picolinate–1000 mg)
- 1 capsule L-Arginine (900 mg)
- 1 capsule Alpha-lipoic Acid (300 mg)
- 4 ounces (1/2 cup) organic whey protein drink (check recipe section)
- 1/2 ounce (1 tablespoon (ACV)–Yoder's Good Health Recipe diluted in 8 ounces of water *

[*Ed.*: We suggest you dilute the ACV. It's an acid and this means it can be hard on the teeth. You can dilute it in 5-8 ounces of water which will reduce that potential problem.]

Lunch:

- 1/2 ounce (1 tablespoon) Yoder's Good Health Recipe diluted in 8 ounces of water
- 4 ounces (1/2 cup) organic whey protein drink

Dinner:

- 2 capsules Albion Chelated Chromium (200 mg each) (Contains Chromium Nicotinate and Glycinate)
- 1 capsule Alpha-lipoic Acid (300 mg)
- 1 capsule L-Arginine (900 mg)
- 1 capsule Gymnema Sylvestre (250-400 mg)
- 1/2 ounce (1 tablespoon) Yoder's Good Health Recipe diluted in 8 ounces of water
- 4 ounces organic whey protein drink

*We sourced these online from *www.swansonvitamins.com* and an article from Reader's Digest[1]. We did not use everything everyone suggested. You may not either. You should consider their advice, but in the end you need to decide for yourself what might work best for you.

Part of the secret of this program is learning what **your** body needs and supplying that need. While the chemistry of our bodies is all basically the same, there may be things that work better for you than others—and other things that work for others, but just don't seem to work for you.

Don't let those challenges keep you from ultimate success. There is an answer for you just like there was for me. Search for it. Hopefully what we have shared with you will be a significant source of that help.

One thing I have learned from my tech-savvy daughters is this: IF you have a question or a problem, "Google" it! Someone else has almost certainly had the same problem—and often found a solution. You can too. Remember, ultimately, you are the only person whose primary job is to look out for you. Stay vigilant.

Chapter 12

Testing and Monitoring Blood Sugar Level

I. Why You Test It

There is no way around this. You have to monitor your blood sugar, and you have to do it often. Why? That's simple. You need to know if your program is working, or if it is not. In fact, the negative information is probably *more* important than the positive.

This may sound surprising, but it's really not. Think about it. How much do you really learn from your successes? Usually not much. But you can learn a tremendous amount from your mistakes if you take the time to analyze where you failed. But success does confirm your program is working—and that **is** important to know.

Why test it so often? Two main reasons: First, because your blood sugar can be very high, yet you feel just fine. You may be sensing something is not quite right, but since you don't know what it is, and it's not really affecting you (or at least you're not aware of it), you may tend to ignore it.

You might feel a little "buzz" when you get a sugar overload, but if it's not painful (which it usually isn't), then you might not feel any concern.

You cannot afford to do this! In this case, you can bank on the fact that ignorance will not lead to bliss.

You need to know what your body is doing, and how it is reacting to your diet and exercise program in real time. This takes regular monitoring. If you convince yourself of the value of this now, it will make it a lot easier. Down the road, especially when you have things under control, it may become tedious. That's a danger zone.

This is the time when the proper understanding of the value of faithfully monitoring your blood sugar will have to kick in and carry you. Diabetes is not a bacterial infection for which you can take 10 days of antibiotics, kill the bug, cure the infection, and then go your way. This is a disease, not an infection.

Diabetes is a systemic physical weakness that you have developed, and will likely have the rest of your life. You may control it; you just can't cure it. As we said in the beginning of the book, you may recover from diabetes, but you will always have to be careful of the weakness you have developed. Life will be a lot easier if you don't try to deny this; just learn to live with it. Things can go haywire, literally, in a couple of days. You **need** to know where you are on a daily basis, and stay in control.

The second reason is that your blood sugar can (and likely will) fluctuate throughout the day—sometimes wildly—and for all kinds of reasons, some good, some not so good. Here's an example.

Do you realize that your blood sugar will rise *every* time you eat? It will. It could rise 30-40 points or it could rise 140 points. It all depends on what, when and how much you are eating. The really important question is whether or not your blood sugar level comes back down in a reasonable amount of time after you eat. More about this later.

II. How Do You Test It?

How do you test blood sugar? The obvious answer is by testing the blood. That's no surprise. The hospital can do it different ways, but there is one option for home testing—and thankfully, it's quite simple. You simply prick the tip of your finger, take a drop of blood and put it on a test strip, and in five to seven seconds you will get a digital readout of your blood sugar level.

The good news is that since diabetes is now a $200+ billion industry, lots of big companies have a vested interest in having you test your blood sugar regularly. They make complete home kits which include a spring-loaded lancet, a digital monitor, and individual test strips.

Even better news is that these kits are both economical and provide a relatively painless blood-testing experience. You can spend more and you will probably get a little more accurate reading, but at the volume of testing we were doing the first three months, we opted for the Walmart option. You know, cheap.

The starter kit we chose is produced by a company called ReliOn (sold at Walmart). The kit is called "Blood Glucose Monitoring System" and sells for about $24.95. It includes a starter supply of both needles (ultra-thin needles called "lancets"), and test strips which slide into the digital monitor (automatically activating it), and calculating your blood glucose level.

You use one lancet and one test strip in each test (you do not want to use the needles multiple times; the infection danger is just not worth the risk for the miniscule savings you might gain). At this writing, a whole box of ReliOn lancets (200+ lancets) is only $9.00, and the test strips are $9.00 for a box of fifty. Of course, you can spend a lot more for similar kits which do the same thing, but this one has done the job nicely for over a year. Again, that choice is yours.

When you consider what things normally cost for medical supplies in most cases, this is a no-brainer. When you break it down, the cost of testing your blood sugar daily is around $5.00

per month. For the first few months it will be a little more than that, since you will be testing it more often.

As you will quickly figure out, this is pretty much the old "razor blade" approach. They are willing to practically give you the test kit so they can sell you the lancets and blood test strips for the rest of your life (and the medicine!). Make no mistake about it, these people know they have a cash cow! But since we have to have it, it's nice that the cost is fairly reasonable; not much else in the medical world is.

III. When Do You Test It?

Opinions will vary on this, but this was our strategy. We wanted to know how my blood sugar fluctuated *throughout* the day. We had researched enough to know that it could fluctuate wildly for many reasons. We decided to take it four times per day until we got it under control. We determined that for me, the goal was to have my blood sugar numbers in the range of 110-120 mg/dl. That was what we considered "under control."

Daily Protocol: I tested my blood sugar four times per day during the first four months, until I was confident that my readings were stable in the 110-125 mg/dl range (below 125 mg/dl is considered pre-diabetic—in other words, standard medical protocol indicates an attempt should be made to address it with diet and exercise and supplements, before resorting to prescription meds).

To reach this goal, I tested first thing in the morning—before I had eaten or drunk anything, other than water—then before lunch, then before dinner, and finally, before I went to bed.

I usually took it while I waited for the coffee to brew. Why so early? We were monitoring what is called the "dawn effect."

What is the "dawn effect"?

Here is the *SimpleGuy Solutions* answer.

We noticed that my blood sugar number was higher in the early morning, just after getting up. We couldn't figure out why? No food had been eaten (Eating always raises blood sugar. This is normal, it is supposed to do that. It is WHAT you eat that determines whether it's going to go up a greater or lesser amount).

Still, the question remained, why is it higher in the morning (when I have not eaten anything) than it was the night before? It did not make sense. So, we did more research. It turns out the answer is quite logical—and quite common. It's just that nobody really has any incentive to tell you the answer.

The Dawn Effect

Your body is an amazing creation. If you have read this far, you realize how deeply we believe that. Most of the time, it operates in an incredibly stable, systematic way, much like we see in creation as a whole. It's not random or chaotic, it is very orderly and stable. This is by design.

The days and nights, the seasons and the tides all operate in a very systematic, scheduled way. This is how the farmer knows when to plant his crops and when to reap his harvest. In the same way our bodies are evidently designed to coordinate with a schedule as well. How so? When it gets dark, we go to bed (or used to—and probably still should!); when it gets light, we get up.

Our bodies respond to being on a schedule. Many describe it as a "biological clock." We can adjust that clock to some extent by personal discipline (or an alarm clock!), but much of it is just "built-in hard-wiring" from the Creator.

In the most simplistic analysis, we could say we are designed to sleep at night, and to be up and about during the day. The darkness of night is most conducive to sleep; daylight is most conducive to productive labor. That's pretty obvious.

Your body understands this as well. It also knows that you will need energy to get up and get going, so it begins to provide that energy in the form of secreting insulin into your bloodstream from the liver, while you are still asleep! Why? It knows that dawn is approaching and it assumes you will be getting up soon! It is supposed to release just enough to keep your blood sugar balanced throughout the night, but in a person with diabetes it doesn't always work so well.

Here's the answer from the **American Diabetes Association**:

What Is the Dawn Phenomenon?

> "All people have the "dawn phenomenon," whether they have diabetes or not. The dawn-phenomenon is a surge of hormones that the body produces daily around 4:00 to 5:00 a.m.
>
> "People with diabetes don't have normal insulin responses to adjust for this, and may see their fasting glucose go up.
>
> "The rise in glucose is mostly because your body is making less insulin and more glucagon (a hormone that increases blood glucose) than it needs. The less insulin made by the pancreas, the more glucagon the pancreas makes as a result. Glucagon signals the liver to break down glycogen into glucose. This is why high fasting blood glucose levels are common in people with type 2 diabetes."[1]

Can you do anything to impact this? Or, at least minimize it? Yes.

Here are some steps that may help:

*Eat dinner earlier in the evening (more time to digest it)

*Go for a walk after dinner (helps promote digestion)

What does this mean to us?

Insulin is supposed to enable the liver to regulate how much glucose to release into the blood to enable us to get up and function (the fact that caffeine is the world's dominant stimulant likely means things aren't working quite right for anybody!) but if the pancreas isn't producing the right amount of insulin or there is insulin resistance in the cells, then blood sugar levels will rise.

Here's the **Mayo Clinic** explanation:

> "The dawn phenomenon, also called the dawn effect, is the term used to describe an abnormal early-morning increase in blood sugar (glucose)—usually between 2 and 8 a.m.—in people with diabetes.
>
> Some researchers believe the natural overnight release of the so-called counter-regulatory hormones—which includes growth hormones, cortisol, glucagon and epinephrine—increases insulin resistance, causing blood sugar to rise. High morning blood sugar may also be caused by insufficient insulin the night before, insufficient medication dosages or carbohydrate snack consumption at bedtime."[2]

Their conclusion is either more meds or cut out late night snacks. Which do you think makes more sense?

How Can You Keep This Under Control?

The only real option is to keep it monitored closely. After a year, this is the one daily check I do. I figure if the early morning reading is good, then the regimen I am on is still working properly.

If the morning reading is up, it's usually because I didn't get any exercise the night before or had too many carbs, or both. So, stay with the program and use the "dawn effect" as a gauge of how well your program is working. Remember, if your numbers are really high, it will take some time to get them down.

Which Finger Do You Test?

First, always test before meals, **not** after meals—(and at least 4 hours after meals). Why? Assuming that you haven't been snacking the two or three hours before your meal, this would be the time when your blood sugar should be the lowest. That may seem obvious, but if you're not familiar with this arena, it may not be obvious at all.

So, which finger do you test? In the end, that decision is up to you. Blood is blood—and you only need a drop. However, since you will be testing it often, you likely want to choose areas where there is more padding, such as the tip of a finger.

I want consistency, so I almost always test on my left hand. I also test on the middle or the index finger. By pricking various spots, the sides near the tip or the tip, I can find lots of spots to test without undue pain or bruising of the tissue. You can easily find a dozen spots on each finger, so you can move the test spot around and avoid damage or pain.

Again, most test kits available today have what would qualify as a *micro-needle.* The lancet makes a miniscule pin prick, so pain should be minimal. [Note: You do *not* have to press hard to initiate the pin prick.]

Let me inject here that you absolutely *can* test the fingers on *either* hand. If you do, just take note of what happens on your blood sugar numbers. The fact is, there are variations in the blood flow in our bodies for all kinds of different reasons, some of which we have no idea why it occurs. I like to minimize those possibilities if I can, so I typically use the same hand now.

One last thing. Again, it will be obvious to most, but it may not occur to some—moisture on the fingers will likely mess up the test reading—usually causing it to read higher, if it reads it at all. Make sure your hands are **clean** and completely **dry** when you take a test.

Chapter 13

Our Daily Schedule and Meal Plan Options

We approached the challenge of getting my blood sugar back into a normal range with the idea that adopting a schedule that was as close to "normal" as possible was probably the wisest strategy. Accordingly, we chose a typical "3 meals-a-day" program. Like most people, we ended up limiting our choices for breakfast and lunch and adding more variety to the dinner options. This served to both simplify and streamline the time we had to spend preparing our meals.

We assumed that most people's schedules, like ours, are largely predetermined by their job and/or family routines. Breakfast needs to be early and fast, lunch needs to be quick and as easy as possible, and dinner can be enjoyed with more leisure and preparation.

Just remember, if you can avoid eating anything after 7:30 p.m., getting your blood sugar under control will be that much easier. Adding a walk or two each day will also be a big plus, even if it's just for ten to fifteen minutes at a time.

Below we have detailed our daily menus for breakfast, lunch, and dinner. We created two options for breakfast, two for lunch and we have listed seven options for dinner.

The breakfast, lunch, and mid-afternoon snack options are the ones we suggest you consider following closely.

The dinner options have more flexibility, depending on your food budget. Those who can afford it may want to include steak (vs. hamburger) or fresh salmon or halibut (vs. flounder). The point is to guide you into providing the right ***balance*** of protein, carbs, and fats along with the ***limited*** portions that will allow your body the nourishment it needs and at the same time lessen the burden of sugar processing so the body can heal itself. Before we give you our suggested meal plans, we need to address one last thing.

Drinks at Meals

Often one of the biggest challenges for diabetics is getting rid of all the sugar drinks we tend to survive on in America—Cokes, diet Cokes (using anything with aspartame is, in our opinion, worse than regular Coke!), and concentrated bottled juices (i.e., anything with high fructose corn syrup (HFCS) as the sweetener) will likely destroy any benefits you get with this program.

Obviously, water is the best choice—and for most people that means filtered or bottled water. Believe it or not, once you get over your sugar addiction (and face it, this IS what it is, an addiction), you will find pure water to be very satisfying. I found it takes about four days to cleanse the system of the physical addiction to sugar, after that it is more a matter of keeping the temptations out of your way (as in dump anything that poses a threat to you staying with the program!).

Having said that, we all know that "variety is the spice of life." I don't know who said that, but having the same thing all the time can get boring—and boredom is a real threat to any restrictive diet program—and this one qualifies. So it was important to provide a little variety wherever we could. We did it with tea.

Slique Tea

Slique Tea (pronounced "sleek") is sold as a slimming diet tea. It is a combination of premium jade oolong tea leaves, ocotea leaves, vanilla essential oil, and Arabian frankincense. My wife is a tea-lover and she loves the oolong tea flavor; lots of people do and for them, this is a great option. I am more of a coffee-person, so I am not that excited about green and white teas (though she did periodically brew some high-end Harney & Sons teas that were quite good.) However, the Slique tea has a component (the ocotea leaves) that evidently have a positive impact on blood sugar. So you get a little bit of the weight control plus the blood sugar aid in this tea. It's marketed by a company called Young Living (which also has some of the highest grade of therapeutic essential oils available.) To order this, you can go to the website or you can just call Beka at (864) 884-9309. Order direct at youngliving.org/rebekahbrazier.

When I drink tea, I like something a little more fruity or minty. Slique tea can be a real asset to diabetics who need weight control support. So, it was important to make this something that we would be glad to drink two to three times per day. We found the solution: Blend it with an herbal tea.

I love the taste of herbal and mint teas. Celestial Seasonings has several "zinger" teas which are herbal (caffeine-free) teas. I use two bags of one of the zinger teas with one or two bags of Slique tea and steep them for about five minutes to make about 1/2 gallon of tea. I can drink all I want.

For a change of pace (and flavor), I will substitute a strong mint or peppermint-flavored tea (Breezy Morning, and Swanson both have great ones) for the zinger. Now I get plenty of fluids and don't have to harass myself to do it! Either one is a great option.

For the meal plans that we followed, these are some samples of what we did for the first three months. Some plans may have specific recipes, but most are a general idea. Try to keep the food as close to its original state as much as possible. We did not do a lot of combination dishes such as casseroles because it tends to increase the carbohydrate intake which we wanted to avoid. We concentrated on steaming, roasting, grilling, and sautéing.

[**Note**: For us, it was essential that we completely prepared our plates with everything we planned to eat in one sitting. We weighed or measured all of our portions and placed all parts of the meal on the plate for a pleasing, colorful (artistic) look. It does make a difference. We did not sample any of it until we sat down to eat. ***Grazing*** *not allowed"*.

[In addition, it was important to *finish* our meal with a small serving of fruit which left us with a wonderful, satisfied feeling. No seconds were allowed. (If you have to, put any left-overs away *before* sitting down to eat so one is not tempted to have seconds).

Breakfast Meal Plan: Option #1

2 whole eggs (fried in butter, scrambled, poached, hard-boiled, etc.)

¼ cup prepared quinoa (served with coconut oil/butter**)

¼ slice 100% whole grain wheat bread* with 1 ½ teaspoon extra virgin coconut oil

2 chicken sausage links or patties without preservatives or nitrates

1 tablespoon *Yoder's Good Health Recipe* Apple Cider Vinegar (ACV) diluted in 5-8 ounces of water.

4 ounces whey (from grass fed sources) protein drink (see chapter 14 for recipe section)

Fresh fruit (See note below for specific portions) ***

4-5 raw almonds, pecans, or walnuts

Breakfast Meal Plan: Option #2

2 ounces homemade rolled oats granola (see recipe section). The benefit of making your own is that you control the sweetening. We used **raw** honey which did not affect my blood sugar.

4-5 ounces of whole milk (non-homogenized, if possible)

1 hard-boiled egg or 2 ounces hard cheese

¼ slice high-quality whole grain bread* with 1-1 ½ teaspoon

extra virgin coconut oil**

1 tablespoon *Yoder's Good Health Recipe* Apple Cider Vinegar (ACV) diluted in 5-8 ounces of water.

4 ounces whey protein drink (from grass-fed sources). See Chapter 14 for recipe section.)

Fresh fruit ***

4-5 raw pecans or almonds or walnuts or cashews, etc.

*Because the amount of bread allowed is so small, it is really imperative that you get as close to a basic freshly-ground whole-grain bread (not a sweet bread) as possible. Either make your own whole grain bread or splurge on some high-quality bread. Remember, you're only eating 1/4 slice!

Whole Foods has good bread and there is also a company called Great Harvest Bread Company which has awesome breads (we used a delicious organic spelt bread, when it was available.) If you have one in your city or nearby, count yourself blessed.

They grind their grain on location and the whole-grain breads are dense and were our choice for this diet. Check with your bread store for possible organic and other grain choices. Also, because we ate such small portions, we could afford to pay more for quality and healthier bread.

** Everywhere coconut oil is mentioned, we specifically mean organic extra virgin cold-pressed coconut oil. It's worth it.

***Focus on fruits in season. To be specific, for a meal my wife served either 4 slices of an apple (about 1/4 of an apple), *or* 4 orange wedges (1/2 orange), *or* 1 ounce of banana sliced, *or* 10 blueberries, 5 grapes, etc.

Lunch Meal Plans

[Note: We wanted a light but satisfying lunch. In order to accomplish this, we had to include some good fats. This was especially important because we were now eating smaller portions, trying to exercise more, and didn't want to have hunger problems.]

We used **four** protein staples to anchor our lunches:

1. Lightly-smoked sardines (bone-in, skin on)
2. Home-made hummus
3. Hard-boiled eggs
4. Cheese wedges (usually hard cheeses, e.g., Cheddar, Swiss, Kerrygold Dubliner, Muenster, and so many more. Experiment!)

As we noted earlier, sardines are not normally a "fan favorite" unless you are already into health food. But let me reiterate that it is as close to a "miracle" food as you are likely to find for type 2 diabetics. Give it a chance.

When I get tired of sardines (which WILL happen), I put one tablespoon of a preferred salad dressing on them, and then put them on crackers. I have used blue cheese dressing, classic French dressing, ranch dressing…use whatever kind you like to overcome any dislike you might have of sardines. The health benefits are worth it.

Here are our suggested lunch ideas, and again, these are only samples of what we did the first three months:

Lunch Meal Plan: Option #1

2 ounces sardines

4-6 flatbread crackers (whole-grain if possible)

4-5 raw veggies (celery sticks, carrot sticks, broccoli, etc.)

½ avocado with tablespoon dressing (French, etc.)

5 raw walnuts (or other raw nuts)

½ tablespoon Yoder's Good Health Recipe (ACV Mix)

Fresh fruit - 4 slices or wedges of ½ apple or 10 blueberries, 6 grapes or 4 orange slices, etc. (in season)

2-4 ounces whey protein milk drink (See recipe in chapter 14)

Lunch Meal Plan: Option #2

2 hard-boiled eggs or 2 ounces cheddar cheese

1 tablespoon home-made hummus

½ cucumber (sliced into spears)

½ tomato (sliced into wedges)

¼ slice 100% whole wheat bread w/1 teaspoon of extra virgin coconut oil

2-4 ounces whey protein drink (See recipe in chapter 14)

4-5 raw nuts

½ cup fresh fruit (See above)

Mid-afternoon Snack

Sometimes you will find yourself wishing you had a snack that won't destroy all the progress you are achieving with the rest of your diet. Since hummus is so good at keeping blood sugar stable, it figures a lot in our afternoon snacks. Here are some good options.

Option #1: 3-4 (or more) cucumber spears with 2 tablespoons of hummus

Option #2: 2-3 cheese slices with 3-4 water crackers and a few apple wedges

Option #3: 3-4 celery stalks with 1-2 tablespoons natural peanut butter*

Option #4: 3-4 apple slices with 2 tablespoons hummus

*[**Note**: There are several nut butters you can use to vary this option.]

Dinner Meal Plans

Dinner Meal Plan: Option #1

Suggested Entree:

4 ounces hamburger with 1 ounce hard cheese (no hamburger buns first 3 months)

Suggested Side Dishes:

½ cup roasted potato (medium diced chunks)*

¾ cup sautéed crisp-tender green beans

⅓-½ cup sliced and roasted red/yellow sweet peppers*

¼ slice whole wheat bread with 1 ½ teaspoons of extra virgin coconut oil. A little raw honey is okay, too.

4 slices of ½ apple (see above recommendations)

5 raw nuts

Drinks:

1 tablespoon Yoder's Good Health Recipe ACV diluted in 5-8 ounces of water

8 ounce glass of iced Slique tea (mixed w/herbal tea, if desired)

3 ounces whey protein drink (See chapter 14 for recipe)

Dessert:

2 Oatmeal Shortbread Cookies (These may also be saved for a light evening snack—no later than 7:30 p.m.)

*Preheat oven to 400°F. Wash all vegetables and dry.

For potatoes (and butternut squash): Dice into 1 inch chunks and place in a bowl. Coat well with extra virgin olive oil, and a pinch of salt (add herbs, if desired), before spreading out in a parchment-lined jelly roll pan or a low-walled broiler pan. Roast in the oven for 30 minutes. Stir and remove when golden brown.

For sweet peppers, remove the seeds and ribs and coat with extra virgin oil and a pinch of salt. Place on a parchment-lined, bottom part of a broiler pan and roast 20 minutes. Stir and remove the vegetables when they are done.

For Brussel sprouts, halve each sprout and toss with extra virgin olive oil. Roast for 20 minutes. Stir and remove when edges are browned.

[**Note**: For salt, we used pink Himalayan salt.]

Dinner Meal Plan: Option #2

Entree:

4 ounces flounder or other light white fish baked with a lime or lemon/garlic/extra virgin oil sauce topped with toasted sliced almonds

Side Dishes:

½ cup of steamed crisp-tender broccoli

¼ cup of cooked brown rice

½ cup coleslaw mixed with slaw dressing (try mixing in walnut oil for a different taste. If you make your own, leave out sugar! Raw honey is okay.)

3 large strawberries

5 raw walnut halves

¼ slice 100% whole wheat/grain bread with extra virgin coconut oil

Drinks:

1 tablespoon Yoder's Good Health Recipe ACV diluted in 5-8 ounces of water.

8 ounces or more iced Slique tea (we mixed ours with a Zinger tea)

3 ounces whey protein drink (see recipe section)

Dessert:

2 Oatmeal Shortbread Cookies (no later than 7:30 p.m.)

Dinner Meal Plan: Option #3

Entree:

4 ounces baked or grilled chicken breast

Side Dishes:

¼ cup cooked quinoa

½ cup roasted Brussel sprouts (see note for roasting vegetables under Dinner Meal Plan: Option #1)

⅓ cup julienned carrots lightly cooked with ginger and honey

½ pear with 1 teaspoon mayo, topped with 1 tablespoon shredded cheddar cheese

¼ slice 100% whole wheat bread with 1-2 teaspoons coconut oil

5 raw cashews

Drinks:

1 tablespoon Yoder's Good Health Recipe AVC diluted in 5-8 ounces of water

3 ounces whey protein drink (See recipe section)

8 ounces or more iced Slique tea (mixed, if desired, with another herbal tea)

Dessert:

2 Oatmeal Shortbread Cookies (no later than 7:30 p.m.)

Dinner Meal Plan: Option #4

Entree:

4 ounces steak (or beef of your choice)

Side Dishes:

½ baked sweet potato with butter

8-10 lightly sautéed asparagus shoots

1 *small* mixed greens salad with 3 grape tomatoes, 7-8 slices of cucumber, ½ green onion chopped, 1/8 cup cheese chunks, etc., with small amount of blue cheese dressing or a freshly made dressing of balsamic vinegar and extra virgin olive oil with herbs and salt and pepper to taste

¼ slice whole wheat bread with 1 teaspoon coconut oil

10 blueberries

5 raw nuts of your choice

Drinks:

1 tablespoon Yoder's Good Health Recipe ACV diluted in 5-8 ounces of water

3 ounces whey protein drink (see recipe in chapter 14)

8 ounce glass of Slique tea (mixed, if desired)

Dessert:

2 Oatmeal Shortbread Cookies (no later than 7:30 p.m.)

Dinner Meal Plan: Option #5

Entree:

1–1 ½ cups of lentil soup with chunks of lamb with a hot sauce,

Or, 1 cup of lentil soup

½ cup of cooked brown rice

Side Dishes:

½ tomato cut in wedges*

½ cucumber sliced*

2 slices of purple onion*

¼ slice 100% whole wheat bread with butter or coconut oil

5 raw pecans

4 slices/wedges of ½ orange

*Tomato, cucumber, and purple onion drizzled with extra virgin olive oil, balsamic vinegar, chopped fresh basil, and salt and pepper to taste. Serve with small sprinkles of cheese such as Feta or Mozzarella or even grated Asiago cheese on top.

Drinks:

1 ounce Yoder's Good Health Recipe ACV diluted in water
3 ounces whey protein drink (See recipe in chapter 14)
8 ounces or more iced Slique tea (mixed with another herbal tea, if desired)

Dessert:

2 Oatmeal Shortbread Cookies (no later than 7:30 p.m.)

Dinner Meal Plan: Option #6

Entree:

4 ounces broiled wild salmon

Side Dishes:

¼ cup quinoa salad (see recipe section)

¼ cup green peas lightly cooked

⅓ cup spaghetti squash, cooked and seasoned with salt and pepper to taste

¼ slice 100% whole wheat bread with butter or extra virgin coconut oil

5 raw almonds

4 slices of ½ peach or other fresh fruit

Drinks:

1 tablespoon Yoder's Good Health Recipe ACV diluted in 5-8 ounces of water

3 ounces whey protein drink (see recipe section)

8 ounces or more iced Slique tea (mixed with another herbal tea, if desired)

Dessert:

2 Oatmeal Shortbread Cookies (no later than 7:30 p.m.)

Dinner Meal Plan: Option #7

Entree:

1-1 ½ cups chicken chili (see recipe section)

6 saltine crackers (if desired)

1-2 tablespoon sour cream or Greek yogurt

Side Dishes:

½ cup coleslaw with dressing (no sugar but can be made with honey)

¼ slice 100% whole wheat bread with butter or extra virgin coconut oil

6-10 grapes

5 raw nuts

Drinks:

1 tablespoon Yoder's Good Health Recipe ACV diluted in 5-8 ounces of water

3 ounces whey protein drink (see recipe section)

8 ounce glass or more of iced Slique tea (mixed with an herbal tea, if desired)

Dessert:

2 Oatmeal Shortbread Cookies (no later than 7:30 p.m.)

Chapter 14

OUR FAVORITE RECIPES

Included in this section are key recipes we have used which allowed us to create a sustainable regimen without feeling we were depriving ourselves of satisfying food.

I would like to make a suggestion; if it is possible, get a good quality, electronic food scale for measuring ingredient and food portions. You will need it. For some of these recipes, your finished product will turn out closer to the intended result if you weigh your ingredients, and you might find yourself becoming a happier cook, especially if "getting it right" is important to you.

Our Favorite Homemade Granola

(Makes about 8 cups. Serving size: 2 ounces.)

1. Preheat the oven to 300°F.

2. Line two jelly roll pans with parchment paper.

3. In a small saucepan, heat the following on **low** heat until it becomes liquid. Do not continue to heat after it has melted.

- **⅓ cup (3 ounces) extra virgin coconut oil**
- **½ cup (168 grams) raw honey**

4. While waiting for the oil and honey mixture to melt, in a large mixing bowl, mix the following well:

- **4 cups [320 grams] *rolled* oats (not quick oats)**
- **1 cup [100 grams] raw sliced almonds**
- **1 cup [112 grams] raw broken pecan pieces**
- **1 cup [135 grams] raw sunflower seeds**
- **1 tablespoon ground cinnamon**
- **1/8 (or less) teaspoon salt**

5. Take the honey/coconut oil mixture off the heat and stir in:

- **½ teaspoon orange flavor or extract**
- **2 teaspoon vanilla extract**

6. Pour all of the wet mixture (honey, oil, flavorings) over the dry mixture of seeds, nuts, oats, cinnamon, and salt, and mix thoroughly.

7. Divide and spread evenly the granola mix between the two parchment-lined baking pans.

8. Bake at 300°F for 10 minutes. Take both pans out and stir well; then return to the oven and let the granola bake for another 10 minutes.

9. Remove the pans from the oven and stir in:

- **1/8 cup dried cranberries.**

10. When completely cooled, store in a cool, dry area. If it takes a while for you to get through your granola, you can store it in a sealed container in the refrigerator to keep it fresh longer

Our Favorite Chicken Chili

(Adapted from an A1 Sweet Hickory Sauce Recipe)

In the last few years Chicken Chili has risen greatly in popularity, and many now prefer it to traditional beef chili. For our purposes, we found it a satisfying alternative for type 2 diabetics. We also found that you can substitute turkey during the holiday/winter season and it's a great fit as well. Many variations will work. For us, this was a great foundation to start on. Makes about 8 cups.]

Mix together the following in a large sauce pan:

- **2 (15 ounce) cans of chili beans, do not drain**
- **2 (10 ounce) can of Rotel mild diced tomatoes and peppers**
- **¼ cup Sweet Hickory A-1 Sauce**
- **3 cups shredded or chopped cooked chicken breast (or turkey)**
- **1 teaspoon Italian seasoning**
- **1 teaspoon "Better Than Chicken Bouillon"**

Bring to a boil in a heavy saucepan, then lower the heat, and let it gently simmer for 30 minutes or longer

Serve with shredded cheese and sour cream as toppings

Makes 8 servings

Our Favorite Whey Protein Recipe

(Makes about 1 ¼ quart of protein drink)

- **93 grams (1 scant cup) Swanson Whey Protein Powder** (basic grass-fed powder with no sweeteners added – follow package directions to make 1 quart)
- **1 heaping tablespoon (15 grams) unsulfured blackstrap molasses** (Golden Barrel is our favorite)
- **1 heaping tablespoon of dark cocoa (or more to taste)**
- **Artificial sweetener to taste**
- **32 ounces (4 cups) non-homogenized whole milk.** (Look for milk that has lower heat pasteurization. We are able to get Mountain Fresh Creamery milk that is pasteurized to 140 degrees, so the good in the milk is not completely destroyed. Also, I believe Whole Foods in some areas may carry other brands of non-homogenized, low-pasteurization milk. If my wife can find it from a good source, she prefers raw milk for health purposes.)

  [**Note**: We *never* used Equal or NutraSweet (aspartame) or Splenda (sucralose), but did use Saccharin (Sweet and Low.) We did a lot of research on artificial sweeteners and determined we did not want to use aspartame or sucralose].

Instructions: Mix all ingredients together and blend well. Chill or serve immediately. Makes about 5 cups of whey protein drink. Good for about 1 week.

Our Favorite Hummus

A friend introduced me to this hummus recipe from the "Inspired Taste" website. It is easy to make, and tastes better than store-bought! Lots of potential for variety in flavor depending upon what you add. Makes about 2 cups.

1. Mix the following in this order:
    - **4 ounces (¼ cup) tahini**
    - **2 ounces (¼ cup) of *fresh* lemon juice**
2. Process for 1 minute in a food processor.
3. Add:
    - **1/2 garlic clove, smashed, and minced**
    - **1/2 teaspoon ground cumin**
    - **1/2 teaspoon Himalayan salt (to taste)**
4. Process for 1 minute more in the food processor
5. Add:
    - **1/2 15 ounce can of chickpeas (garbanzo beans), drained and rinsed**
6. Process for one minute
7. Add:
    - **½ (remainder of) can of chickpeas**
8. Process until mixture is smooth and spreadable.
9. Add while processing:
    - **1-2 tablespoons water (to aid in smoothing)**

To serve: Drizzle extra virgin olive oil on top.

Optional: Add ¼ teaspoon of ground chipotle pepper or Paprika or add some *finely* chopped nuts, for variety.

To Serve: Scrape the hummus into a bowl then drizzle about 1 tablespoon of olive oil over the top and sprinkle with paprika. Serve with crackers or cut vegetables.

To Store: Store homemade hummus in an airtight container and refrigerate up to one week.

*Tahini is a paste of ground sesame seeds. *Krinos* is the best-tasting store-bought brand we have found. It's available in many grocery stores.

Oatmeal Shortbread Cookies

(Makes around 40 cookies)

For these cookies, my wife likes to weigh out the recipe ingredients, so in this list, the grams are exact, but the "cups" are nearly exact. If you have an electronic food scale, now is the time to pull it out.

[**Note:** Once the cookie dough is put together, it should be allowed to chill in the refrigerator for at least 4-5 hours or overnight before baking.]

1. Mix together in a large mixing bowl until soft and creamy:
   - **50 grams (¼ cup packed) light brown sugar**
   - **50 grams (¼ cup less 1 ½ teaspoons) organic cane sugar**
   - **5 ounces (10 tablespoons) unsalted butter softened**
   - **1 ounce (2 tablespoons) extra virgin coconut oil**
2. Mix together in a small bowl:
   - **¼ cup of grated apple, peeled and seeds removed (or you can use ¼ cup of unsweetened apple sauce)**
   - **1 teaspoon of vanilla extract**
   - **½ teaspoon of orange flavoring or extract**
3. Add the grated apple, orange flavoring, and vanilla extract to the sugars, butter, and coconut oil and beat together well.
4. In another bowl, mix together the following dry ingredients and set aside:

- **80 grams (1/2 cup plus 1 tablespoon) whole grain flour***
- **100 grams (3/4 cup plus 1 tablespoon) King Arthur cake flour**
- **1 teaspoon Himalayan salt (or sea salt, if you have it)**
- **120 grams (1 cup plus 3 tablespoons) quick cooking oats**

5. Set the mixer on a slow speed and slowly spoon in the dry flour/oat mixture, blending well after each addition until smooth.

6. Form into 2 6-inch long rolls about 2 in. diameter and wrap in plastic. Refrigerate 4-5 hours.

7. When ready to bake, preheat the oven to 300°F.

8. Place parchment paper on a cookie sheet, remove one cookie dough roll from the refrigerator and slice into ¼ in. slices and place on the parchment covered cookie sheet.

9. Bake the cookies for 18-20 minutes or until barely golden brown around the edges. Remove from the oven and let cool for 1 minute on the cookie sheet, then place on a rack till completely cool.

10. Store in an air-tight container. Serving portion: 2 cookies.

*Note: I purchase organic kamut berries from an excellent source for natural food (www.breadbeckers.com), and grind my own flour (fine). Kamut flour has a mild flavor and works well for this recipe. You can use spelt or whole wheat flour if you can't find kamut grain or flour.

Favorite Quinoa Options

Quinoa is one of the most adaptable, delicious, and nutritious grains known to man. It can be served hot as a rice alternative or cold as a middle-eastern tabbouleh-like dish. (Though it tastes much like a Mediterranean dish, it is actually derived from the Andean mountain regions of South America).

It is delicious either way it is served. We like to make as large a batch as possible, use some as a brown rice substitute, and then make the rest into a delicious cold quinoa salad.

To prepare: (Makes about 3 cups)
In a medium sauce pan, bring to a boil:

- **2 cups water**
- **¼ teaspoon salt**

Add to the boiling water:

- **1 cup quinoa, rinsed well and drained**

Bring to a boil over high heat, then turn down the heat and simmer 15 minutes until the liquid is absorbed. Turn off heat and let sit 5 minutes. Fluff with a fork before serving.

Serve hot as a rice substitute with butter or coconut oil and/or broth as desired. Salt and pepper to taste.

Cold Quinoa Salad Options

Creating a great cold quinoa salad is simply a matter of adding the ingredients to create a flavor you like. Be creative! Here is one idea that worked well for us:

Stir together:

- **2 cups cooked, cold quinoa**
- **¼ cup chopped green onion**
- **¼ cup chopped purple onion**
- **2 medium-diced tomatoes**
- **½ cup chopped cucumber**
- **1-2 tablespoons chopped fresh basil**
- **⅓ cup Feta cheese crumbles**

For the dressing, mix together:

- **zest of ½ lemon**
- **¼ cup extra virgin olive oil**
- **¼ cup fresh lemon juice**
- **½ teaspoon sea salt**

Toss the quinoa, onions, tomatoes, cucumber, and Feta cheese together with the dressing. Chill for 1 hour before serving.

Serving Size: ½ cup

[Note: Other options, additions **or** substitutions are listed below. You can add or vary the amounts and types of ingredients according to your liking or taste.]

For example:

- ⅓ cup broken pecan pieces
- 1-2 tablespoons mint leaves chopped fine (substitute for the basil)
- ⅓ cup cranberries
- ½ cup of chopped apple (substitute for tomatoes)

BONUS PREVIEWS

OF *COMING* SIMPLEGUY SOLUTIONS℠ BOOKS

BONUS PREVIEW #1

The Rx Drug Survival Information Kit

How to Use Your DNA to Survive
In the Deadly World of Rx Drugs

BONUS PREVIEW #2

"29 Home Remedies...that Work!"

Learn about the *Thieves Advantage*—

Essential Oils That Survived the Plague!

...and still work in today's sick world.

*These statements have not been evaluated by the Food and Drug Administration. These products are not intended to diagnose, treat, cure or prevent any disease. Always consult your physician if you have any questions.

Bonus Preview #1

"THE Rx DRUG SURVIVAL INFORMATION KIT"

HOW PERSONALIZED MEDICINE USES YOUR DNA TO HELP YOU SURVIVE IN THE DEADLY WORLD OF PRESCRIPTION DRUGS

Preview

Imagine a world in which a 747 jetliner crashes, not somewhere else in the world, but somewhere in America—every day—and every soul on board dies. No survivors. None. Everyone dies. This means over 100,000 people would die...every year!

Now imagine in the same world, each day another *fifteen* 747 jets crash every day, only these passengers don't die, they just end up hospitalized. That would mean over two *million* people would end up hospitalized...every year. Some with injuries from which it may take years to recover.

Sound bizarre? Hard to imagine? Think that it could not possibly happen here? Sorry to have to be the bearer of bad tidings—it is already happening. Welcome to the real world—today's world of Rx (Prescription) Drugs. You already live there.

Of course, we all know that if an event like crashing jets were to actually occur in America all the airlines would immediately ground their entire fleets.

Service would be discontinued until a solution was found. Such a crisis would **never** be allowed to continue. It would be unthinkable. 9/11/2001 proved that.

But in the world of pharmaceutical medicine it happens every year. Sadly they are considered "acceptable losses." The crashing jets illustration was first coined by Dr. Peter Dimitri, a former Assistant Surgeon General for the Air Force and the only officer ever to be both a test pilot and also a medical doctor in the Air Force. He wanted to bring some real world perspective to the crisis we are confronted with in the ongoing epidemic of tragic adverse drug reactions.

Those numbers are not imaginary. They are hard facts. In this country over one hundred thousand people die each year because of adverse drug reactions (ADRs). Another two to four *million* end up in the hospital...each and every year.

Millions more have adverse drug reactions, but are never reported since they are not severe enough to require hospitalization. The amazing fact is that over 90% of these adverse drug reactions (ADR's) are avoidable. They need not happen.

How Can This Be True?

Adverse drug reactions are now the **fourth** leading cause of death in America. Yet, if you look at the United States Center for Disease Control's (CDC) annual list of the leading causes of death, it is not even listed. You find the usual suspects: cancer, heart disease, acute respiratory distress, influenza, etc. But *adverse drug reactions* (ADRs) are not even listed. You have to go to the United States Food and Drug Administration (FDA) to find out the truth. Just search the Web for *FDA ADR Statistics* and see for yourself.

You probably know someone (or maybe you yourself) who has experienced an adverse drug reaction. Why is it treated with such complacency? Why are we not more aware of it? Why is it allowed to continue?

The answer is two-fold. The first part is ignorance; the second part is medical reality. The ignorance is on our part. We simply are unaware that now there *is* a solution. The second part is the medical reality that, up until now, there was no solution. Doctors were simply doing the best they could with the information they had. This is the way medicine is really practiced.

Trial and Error Medicine

When a doctor puts out his shingle to start his business, what does he call it? He calls it a *practice*. There is a good reason.

It comes as a shock to many to find out that much of our beloved mainstream clinical medicine is based on guesswork, very highly-educated guesswork, to be sure—but guesswork nevertheless. In the everyday world, we normally call it a trial-and-error approach. How does it work?

We think we know the best approach to solving a problem, based on all the current knowledge and experience we have, so we try it. If it doesn't work, then we try something else. We keep doing it until we find something that works. However, sometimes the things that do not work can cause serious problems.

You might be asking, "How can doctors do this? Why don't they know what will work?" Up until now, there really was no way for them to know how a particular individual would react to their prescribed treatment. They used their best judgment, a combination of skill, experience, and education. They also are forced to heavily rely on pharmaceutical research.

Before a pharmaceutical company manufactures a drug, all kinds of testing is done to determine and prove two things: first, does it work; second, does it do any harm. If so, how much? Do the benefits outweigh the harm done? If so, it gets FDA approval.

So why did they prescribe it? Because, based on the test results, most people seemed to do well. What that means is: the benefits of the majority seemed to outweigh the risk of harm to the minority who had adverse reactions. Usually, many more people seemed to be helped than harmed.

This is also the justification for those staggering statistics we began with. If you are asking yourself the question, How can over a hundred thousand people dying each year and millions ending up in the hospital for adverse drug reactions ever be considered "acceptable losses"? The answer is simply that the benefits to millions of others seemed to be worth the risk. The unvarnished truth is that it's very much like a lottery, only in reverse. Until now there was no way to predict who the winners and losers would be.

But in the clinical situation (i.e. where you are meeting face-to-face with your personal doctor), most doctors are still treating you based on the assumption that you will react like most other people to his prescribed treatment. He is still relying on the hope that you will react like most other people to the Rx drugs.

But as we all know, we are *not* like other people, we are unique—we are all different. Yet while the doctor might have seen us as unique individuals, he really didn't have the tools to treat us as individuals.

This all changed on April 14, 2003.

This was the day that the National Human Genome Research Institute (NHGRI) announced the successful completion of *The Human Genome Project.*

The goal of this project was to sequence a whole human genome (i.e. identify and complete a full analysis of the DNA of a real human being). It was a massive 10-year, $3 billion project. But it began a new era in medicine, the era of what is now being called *Personalized* Medicine.

The Era of Personalized Medicine

> You are the only you God made...God made you and then broke the mold.
>
> – **Max Lucado, *Cure for the Common Life: Living in Your Sweet Spot***

Max Lucado's quote, we believe, is entirely correct. We can also add that God did not break the mold out of frustration, thinking He didn't get it quite right with you! He broke it because He was delighted with what He produced. Our individual uniqueness is simply powerful proof of His truly infinite creativity.

But until now, that has not done us much good when we go to the average doctor's office. But now we have scientific confirmation; it's an incontrovertible fact, there is only one of you. Others may be like you, but they are not *exactly* like you. You are unique, your DNA proves it. But most doctors are still treating you like you are like everyone else. Why?

Please don't misunderstand what I am saying. Most doctors do their very best to treat us with care and concern and give us the best treatment or therapy they possibly can. But until now, they have not had the tools they need to precisely customize medical treatment to each of us individually, to offer what is now very accurately being described as *personalized* medicine.

With the advent of DNA testing for ADRs they can. However, many still do not know it is available and no longer prohibitively expensive.

This is where you will have to be prepared to help your doctor help you. This is what the ***Rx Drug Survival Kit*** will enable you to do—use your DNA to help you survive in the world of prescription drugs.

Tomorrow's Medicine is Here Today!

What is the promise here? And what exactly is "*personalized* medicine"? And does it really make a difference?

Absolutely! It can make an enormous difference in your future, maybe a life and death difference. Here is the story...

In 1993 a scientific project was begun to "sequence" the entire human genome. In layman's terms, the goal was to discover how all of the genes in our body work together. It was an amazing undertaking, it took 10 years to finish and cost over $3 billion dollars. In April 2003 the project which is known as the Human Genome Project was completed.

Whenever you hear the term, DNA testing or whole genome sequencing, this is what it is referring to.

There are scores of companies, large and small, that are now focused on researching DNA testing to find cures for everything from cancer (of which there are more than 100 kinds) to heart disease, diabetes, and drug addictions. It is a field filled with great hope and possibilities and, of course, enormous profits for those who succeed.

The truth is, the fruits of those labors are a long way off...and many will likely *never* bear fruit.

But there is one specific area in which we know we can succeed and have an impact...and do it now! We can now virtually *eliminate adverse drug reactions* and protect you and your family from the tragedies so many are suffering.

The test is called a *pharmaco-genetic* test (PGx test, for short). It is not an invasive test; it only requires a cheek swab for the laboratory analysis. It is quick and painless. But your doctor must be the one to order it. If it's so simple, why can't you go into your local lab and order it?

For some reason the FDA considers a DNA test to be a "medical device" for regulatory purposes...hence, a doctor must order the test. And, since most primary care doctors are not using this tool yet, you will likely have to request it.

We will soon be coming out with a book which details all of these exciting developments. But if you want to get ahead of the curve and act now to protect yourself and your family...all you need is the ***Rx Drug Survival Kit.***

The kit will give you all the basic information you need, plus the essential "Letter of Request to Your Doctor." It will also answer most of the potential questions or resistance you might face if your doctor is unfamiliar with the test.

The complete cost for the *Rx Drug Survival Kit* info kit is only $3.99. Why not $29 or $39 dollars? It's simple. We want you to value us as a trusted source for reliable, solid, actionable health information. It's that simple.

Millions of Americans are being hospitalized each year for adverse reactions to Rx drugs...over 100,000 a year are dying. It's costing insurance companies and the government (us!) over $136 billion in unnecessary expenses. Why? Many doctors just don't know the test is available for clinical use. We can change that. You can help...and in the process you can protect yourself and your family from senseless, needless tragedy.

A very wise man once said that if you're sitting around a table of gamblers and you don't know who the fool is, then you are the fool. We don't want you to be the fool when it comes to taking prescription drugs.

You may not be able to avoid taking the drugs, but you can know if it is the right drug for you! You don't have to accept a lottery ticket when it comes to your health.

But you have to act now to protect yourself and your family. You can help your doctor help you. He will be the wiser...and so will you!

It's now available as an e-book on Amazon.com

Title: *The Rx Drug Survival Information Kit*

Bonus Preview #2

The *Thieves* Advantage

For every drug that benefits a patient, there is a natural substance that can achieve the same effect.

–Pfeiffer's Law, Dr. Carl C. Pfeiffer, M.D.

The art of medicine consists in amusing the patient while nature cures the disease.

–Voltaire, 18th century French Philosopher

Don't you just love it when someone cuts through all the peripheral niceties and strikes at the heart of an issue—totally unconcerned with those on whose toes he steps! During the 18th century French Enlightenment, that sort of courage could cost you your head, literally! But the famous French philosopher Voltaire was such a man. The point is, he makes you think. Could he be right about medicine?

When we think of "mainstream medicine," we often find ourselves in a position where doctors view us as helpless—as if the idea that we could possibly take care of ourselves is either ridiculous or negligent—or maybe both.

With all the almost miraculous medical advances, somehow we have all of a sudden supposedly become helpless. How could we ever have survived without doctors? But we did.

The truth is many people have been taking good care of themselves for a long, long time. As Dr. Pfeiffer's Law suggests, nature has provided cures for almost every illness and ailment we have and many of them are simple, easy to access, readily available, and very economical (which is one reason you do not hear much about them; you can't make much profit selling them—certainly not the kind of profits that pharmaceutical companies can make selling patented drugs!).

Today we call them "Home Remedies." The rise of modern medicine has left an impression that these remedies are no longer effective. This is simply not true...and in these days of growing concern over MRSA and other antibiotic-resistant "bugs," it is becoming more and more important to know about them.

But Voltaire's point is still valid (even if stated a little more harshly than necessary!). Much of mainstream medicine focuses on treating the symptoms of disease, rather than the source of the disease. Usually those symptoms involve pain and/or discomfort of some sort and we expect the doctor to use his "magic" to relieve this discomfort. His magic usually amounts to prescribing a pill.

The real problem here is that we tend to equate eliminating or relieving our discomfort with curing the real problem. While this is understandable, it may not be accurate at all, in fact, it rarely is. The doctor knows this. What he doesn't tell you is that while he may not know the specific cause of your illness, he does have a general idea (i.e., it's some sort of a "bug"), and he knows that if he can relieve or start the process of relieving the discomfort, in a week or two the sickness will run its course and the body will heal itself.

So, the doctor did solve your problem (discomfort), just not the way you thought he did. But as Voltaire noted, you were "amused" long enough for the body to heal itself.

We thought this whole approach to healing and medicine was changing with the advent of molecular medicine and antibiotics. For a time, it seemed like it was working. But unfortunately, many of those dreams of lasting cures have yet to materialize. In fact, some of the problems antibiotics have created are downright scary!

The Advent of Antibiotics

The discovery of antibiotics is usually attributed to a Dr. Alexander Fleming in the 1920's. Like many life-changing discoveries, it was an accident. His discovery was a mold that appeared to kill bacteria. Bacteria are the main cause of infection. Left untreated, bacterial infection can grow until it kills the host. But it was 10 more years before Fleming's work became really useful.

In the late 1930's, London Doctors Howard Florey and Ernst Chain were able to identify and isolate the substance in the mold which killed bacteria. We know it as penicillin.

The important point for us to note is that penicillin is a natural substance—a natural substance which kills bacteria—the bacteria which causes infection. The reputation for its ability to cure infection was permanently established during the D-Day assault on Europe. Multitudes of lives were saved during World War II because the natural "miracle drug" we know as penicillin was able to be mass-produced.

In the 1950s–1960s, antibiotics were all the rage. When you went to the doctor, you expected him to prescribe this new wonder drug which would make you healthy again—and usually it did.

But there were problems lurking with this strategy. Some people turned out to be allergic to penicillin and it had a few nasty side-effects that made it impossible for them to take it.

Ultimately, other "miracle" drugs were developed to take the place of penicillin. As the world of pharmaceutically-created drugs evolved and new drugs were developed. Very few were natural—most were chemical derivatives. This meant they were now patentable, relatively cheap to produce, and able to be sold for exorbitant profits.

But an even bigger problem emerged as doctors realized that the bacteria were alive and reacting to the killing effects of the antibiotics by mutating and developing their own resistance to its killing effects. This was like a science fiction movie coming to life!

Additionally, people were also beginning to realize that one of the side effects of these "miracle" antibiotics was that they tended to wipe out the good bacteria at the same time they killed the disease-causing bacteria. In effect, this left the patient's immune system basically defenseless until the good bacteria could be re-populated in the gut (which is where most of our disease battles are fought).

While you can effectively re-populate the gut with good bacteria through probiotics, it still takes times to establish them. What is needed is a natural alternative, one that can kill bacteria without wiping out the health-supporting bacteria.

Is there such a thing? Not really. Today, some drugs can target certain "bugs" while not harming others, but the damage to the intestinal flora is still significant, so it is essential that we be proactive with the probiotics. Why? The CDC (United States Centers for Disease Control) estimates that about 57,000 people will die this year from influenza and flu-related illnesses! Some flu "bugs" are bacterial and some are viral—often the doctor won't know which it is without testing.

When it comes to illness there is no question that your best defense is a good offense.

If you can protect yourself from getting sick in the first place (by developing a strong disease-resistant immune system), you are way ahead of most people. Here are two products which can give you serious support in your efforts.

The *Thieves* Advantage

In the 14th century, the bubonic plague swept through Western Europe and decimated the population. Estimates of upwards of 20 million deaths are common; worldwide, it may have been as high as 200 million. The impact was truly devastating—economically, socially and financially. But where one person sees a crisis, another sees an opportunity.

The story is told about a small band of thieves in France who realized that no one wanted to go near anyone who died of the plague. You had to pay someone to carry off the bodies. Nobody wanted to touch them.

Many times whole families died within two to three days. Industrious thieves saw this as an opportunity to rob the families of those who had died. Eventually, they were caught.

The citizenry was outraged that these thieves were taking advantage of these families, but what the ruling officials were even more interested in knowing was why they were not catching the disease! The disease was extremely contagious and there was no known natural immunity. Yet for all practical purposes, these thieves seemed to be immune. What was their secret?

In return for leniency in their punishment, they agreed to share the formula they used. The secret turned out to be a blend of aromatic essential oils that (modern science has verified) are both strongly antibacterial and antiviral. They would coat themselves with this blend of oils and protect themselves from the plague.

More recently, one company (*YoungLiving* Essential Oils) has manufactured this essential oil blend (using only the highest quality, therapeutic-grade oils) using this ancient formula. They then had it independently tested at Weber State University in Ogden, Utah to determine its anti-microbial properties. The *Thieves* Essential oil blend was found to have a 99.96% "kill rate" vs. airborne bacteria!*

The amazing part is that it is totally natural. It is a blend of five therapeutic-grade essential oils—clove oil, cinnamon bark oil, lemon oil, rosemary oil and eucalyptus radiata oil.

Taken together, the *Thieves* essential oil blend offers one of the most powerful, natural, immune system-enhancing, respiratory-disease fighting oils found anywhere. As we will outline in the coming book, there are literally over 100 uses for this product—from attacking sore throats to wiping out mold to sanitizing kitchen counters of unwanted bacteria.

If you would like to see some additional, very basic, independent experiments using Thieves oil, look at this—

Biochemist Doctor Annie Pryor (Ph.D., Ohio State University) has done some very interesting work (comparing all kinds of commercially available products). She does not sell any of the products she tests, she merely does basic testing on products people want to have tested. The link for Dr. Annie Pryor, www.stopthestomachflu.com

If you would like to try the Thieves oil blend, here is the link, https://www.youngliving.org/Beka

For questions, contact Beka at (864) 884-9309,

What about an oral supplement? If you would like to have the benefits of the Thieves oil in an oral supplement rather than an oil, you can. *Young Living* has put the Thieves oil blend together with two other really potent herbal additives: Oregano and Thyme. It's a powerful combination. It's called ***Inner Defense***.

Wild oregano (Origanum vulgare) has become increasingly popular in recent years...and for good reason. A team of UK and Indian researchers ran tests and found that Himalayan

Oregano oil was more effective at killing MRSA than 18 other antibiotics. That is impressive for a natural product. [http://www.medicalnewstoday.com/articles/130620.php]

Young Living has put all these potent, immune-enhancing herbs and oils in this powerful **Inner Defense** product. If you want to go on offense against sickness and disease (especially during cold, flu, and allergy season), you should consider **Inner Defense**.

If you would like to try Thieves oil or Inner Defense, you can order it at: www.youngliving.org/Beka

For questions, contact Beka (864) 884-9309.

*Weber State Thieves Test results: (Source: Journal of Essential Oil Research [J. Essent. Oil Res.] Vol. 10, no 5, pp.517-523. Sept-Oct 1998. Weber State University, Ogden, UT)

APPENDIX

Details on the "Cost-Sharing" Healthcare Program Alternative to Obamacare

If you have landed on this page, it's because you wanted more detailed information on the CHM "cost-sharing" healthcare program I referred to at the beginning of this book.

There is no hype in what you have read—or what you will read. I know because I have personally been involved with this group for over 10 years. It is a conservative Christian group with tens of thousands of members who have joined together to share the burden of healthcare costs and have found that they can maintain control of their healthcare choices, yet dramatically reduce their personal cost by joining others who have similar values and lifestyles. It has been successfully operating for over 30 years.

With tens of thousands now participating in this cost-sharing program...and the scary prospect of ObamaCare and the problems it is creating for so many, multitudes are being forced to look for a viable, economical alternative. That's what happened to us over ten years ago when we decided we couldn't afford to educate our children ***and*** pay the high cost of traditional healthcare insurance, so we began to search for a safe, sane alternative. Christian Healthcare was our solution.

How It Works

How does this program work? It's actually quite simple. The program itself is designed to help its members avoid the financial disaster that a serious medical illness or its treatment could potentially wreak on our lives. The focus is on coverage for *major* medical incidents which require hospital care and treatment. It's really ***not*** designed for folks who want to run to the doctor to get a prescription drug every time they get a cough or cold…and want "insurance" to pay for it. In this program, you pay for those visits yourself (which usually means you don't go unless you *really* need to…in which case you're glad to pay for it!). If this is you, read on…

What You Get

The program administrators have designed the program with three levels of coverage (bronze, silver, gold). At this writing (2016) the monthly cost is $45-$85-$150 per person, depending upon what level you choose to participate. The CHM website will give you details regarding what is covered at each level and explain the process of how your healthcare bills are shared and paid. The CHM staff are very knowledgeable and amazingly helpful. This is a ministry to them, not a business. So what are your options?

You choose the level you want based on two criteria: First, how much "coverage" do you want? Do you want just the in-patient and out-patient hospital/doctor expenses related to a major medical event covered? If so, then either the "Bronze" or "Silver" levels might meet your needs.

However, if you want doctor's office visits, Rx drugs, and tests related to the incident, plus all in-hospital and doctor-related expenses, as well as things like home-healthcare, physical therapy and other follow-up services for a period of time after hospitalization…then the "Gold" level will be more attractive.

The second criteria is related to the first. After choosing your desired coverage level, you must determine how much upfront, "out-of-pocket" costs you are willing to be personally responsible for. It's the same idea as the "deductible" portion in traditional insurance. It's the amount you pay "out-of-pocket" before your expenses become eligible for "sharing" with the group.

Here's an example.
At the Bronze level ($45/mo. PP), you are personally responsible for the first $5,000 of incident-related expenses, after which your bills become eligible for "sharing" with the other members.

At the Silver level, you take care of the first $1,000 of expenses, then the rest are eligible for "sharing." (Also, there is **no** traditional "80/20" element where you get stuck with 20% of a huge bill. Once eligible for sharing, all costs are covered up to the program limits—which are quite generous—for the qualified expenses). At the Gold level, you take care of the first $500, then the rest are "shared."

What It Costs

If you're interested so far, then this is really going to get exciting. The monthly cost (which is technically designated a "gift" to the program) is based on your choice of participation level. Each individual person counts as a "unit" (including children). Parents and children all cost the same. But, here is the exciting feature for families—no family pays for more than 3 units. Even if you have four kids, plus two parents, you still only pay for 3 units per family. That's usually a huge savings!

At the lowest level, Bronze, the monthly cost is just $45 per unit. At the silver level, the cost is $85 per unit. At the highest level, Gold, the cost is $150 per unit. I have participated at the Silver level for over ten years and the monthly amount has only been increased one time, from $75 to $85 per unit. This is a real testimony to the kind of management and commitment this group has to the program.

An Example

Let's assume you have a wife and three children. You decide you would like to participate at the Silver level (where you cover the first $1000 of upfront expenses). Your monthly contribution would be based on $85 per "unit." In this example, this would mean 5 units (2 adults and 3 children). Normally, this would mean that you would multiply 5 x $85 (or $425). However, remember there is a ‘cap’ on the ‘per family’ cost of the program—no family is charged for more than 3 units—no matter how many children you have!

This means that when you calculate your contribution, the amount is only $255, not $425! I have friends who have joined the program with 5-7 children; they still pay for only 3 units, but all the children are included! At the Gold level, even maternity benefits/expenses are included.

Again, I want to reiterate this is *not* considered insurance. It is a "cost-sharing" program that is supported by people who have similar values and lifestyles, that's how you qualify. What does this mean in practical terms? It means that you don't have an absolute guarantee that your bills can be paid. If everyone stopped contributing, you would be in the same situation as anyone else who couldn't afford medical insurance. You are ultimately the responsible person. Of course, it also means that you have almost 30 years of history and over 100,000 folks who have had their medical bills shared and paid for a long, long time, without fail. It was a pretty simple decision for us and we've been totally satisfied—and so have all the folks we've referred.

ObamaCare Impact

The best news is that ObamaCare will have no effect on this program. We have been specifically exempted and deemed to have fulfilled the healthcare insurance requirement and, therefore, incur no penalty for not having health insurance. This is truly a win-win program.

If you think this program might be for you, here's the link with all the details and sign-up forms. Once you've signed up, send us an email and we'll show you how to reduce your monthly expense even more.

Don't delay. This is an opportunity you don't want to miss! Questions? Email us at equity1st@yahoo.com. If you want to talk directly with someone at the program or order a complete information package, call (800)791-6225. You can also get all your FAQ questions answered online at www.chministries.org.

FootNotes

DISCLAIMER: We have made every effort possible to verify the accuracy of the sites and links listed below. However, we cannot be held responsible for links that have been discontinued, or otherwise compromised.

Chapter 1

1. www.nlm.nih.gov/medlineplus/ency/article000313.htm

Chapter 2

1. See diabetes.org/diabetes-basic/statistics
2. See cdc.gov/nchs/fastats/leading-causes-of-death
3. See diabetes.org/diabetes-basic/statistics
4. Ibid.
5. Ibid.
6. Ibid.
7. Ibid

Chapter 3

1. www.mayoclinic.org/drugs-supplements/metformin-oral-route/side-effects/drg-20067074

2. www.diabetesincontrol.com/contact-us/6740-new-information-on-how-metformin-works

3. www.mayoclinic.org/drugs-supplements/metformin-oral-route/side-effects/drg-20067074

4. www.mayoclinic.org/diseases-conditions/type-2diabetes/in-depth/diabetes-treatment/art-20051004?pg=2

Chapter 5

1. See livescience.com/3186-brain-food-eat-smart

2. See diabetes.org/food-and-fitness/food/what-can-i-eat/making-healthy-food-choices/fats-and-diabetes

3. See brainyquote.com/quotes/quotes/a/alberteins148866

4. NIH Medline Plus article: What do fats do in the body? (www.medlineplus.gov)

5. Ibid

6. See medicalnewstoday.com/articles/278164.php

7. See FDA.gov/ForConsumers/consumerupdates/ucm293330

8. Find this info and more at: American Heart Association's official site: www.heart.org/HEARTORG/Conditions/More/Diabetes

9. See nlm.nih.gov/medlineplus/ency/imagepages/19514.htm

10. See heart.org/HEARTORG/Conditions/More/Diabetes

11. Ibid.

12 See authoritynutrition.com/healthy-cooking-oils

Chapter 6

1. See the following article at heart.org:

.heart.org/HEARTORG/Conditions/More/MyHeartandStrokeNews/Inflammation-and-Heart-Disease_UCM_432150Article.jsp

2. www.meandmybod.com; topic: anti-inflammatory diets

3. The Complete Idiot's Guide to The Anti-Inflammation Diet (Penguin Group (USA) Inc., 375 Hudson Street, New York, NY, 10014) Copyright 2014 Penguin Group (USA) Inc.

Chapter 7

1. Here's the link to the whole article if you would like to read it:

http://care.diabetesjournals.org/content/27/11/2741.full

2. http://drhyman.com/blog/2014/12/18/7-ways-reverse-obesity-diabetes

3. *Ed*: For an excellent article on magnesium, see

http://drhyman.com/blog/2010/05/20/magnesium-the-most-powerful-relaxation-mineral-available/

Chapter 8

1. www.webmd.com/vitamins-supplements/arginine

2. http://news.ku.dk/all_news/2013/2013.9/amino-acid-with-promising-anti-diabetic-effects/

3. http://www.pmrf.org/projects/larginine.pdf

4. For more info on Alpha Lipoic Acid (ALA) see: WebMD.com

5. For more info on gymnema sylvestre at—WebMD.com

6. For more info cinnamon, see: WebMD.com

7. http://drhyman.com/blog/2012/03/01/time-for-an-oil-change/

8. http://www.goodfats101.com/fats-101/omega09s/

Chapter 9

1. See: http://patients.gi.org/topics/probiotics-for-the-treatment-of-adult-gastrointestianl-disorders/

See also: http://www.medscape.com/viewarticle/770468

2. http//www.gastro.org/info_for-patients/2013/6/6/probiotics

3. http://healio.com/

Search: What are enzymes?

4. https://www.niddk.nih.gov/health-information/health-statistics/Pages/digestive-diseases-statistics-for-the-united-states.aspx#11

5. www.chucklinggoat.co.uk

Chapter 10.

1. www.webmd.com/diet/obesity/apple-cider-vinegar-and-health

2. Ibid.

3. Ibid.

4. http://www.swansonvitamins.com/blog/jenessa/apple-cider-vinegar-uses

http://www.newsmax.com/FastFeatures/apple-cider-vinegar-blood-sugar/2015/09/14/id/691415/

5. Ibid.

6. www.doctoroz.com/slideshow/surprising-ways-use-apple-cider-vinegar

7. www.swansonvitamins.com/blog/jenessa/apple-cider-vinegar-uses

8. bragg.com/products/bragg-organic-apple-cider-vinegar.html

9. Ibid.

10. http://www.swansonvitamins.com/blog/vitamins-supplements-faqs/is-coconut-oil-good-or-bad-for-a-person

11. http://webmd.com/diet/guide/high-protein-low-carbohydrate-diets

12. www.webmd.com/search/2/results?query=protein%diet

13. http://proteinpowder.mercola.com/Miracle-Whey-Protein.html

14. http://www.webmd.com/vitamins-supplements/ingredientmono-901-black%20seed.aspx?activeingredientid=901&activeingredientname=black%20seed

15. PubMedLink: [PMID: 16275613]

16. http://healthimpactnews.com/2014/black-seed-oil-cures-many-cancers-according-to-numerous-studies/

17. http://www.myblackseed.com

Chapter 11

1. The Reader's Digest article was found at:

http://www.rd.com/health/wellness/the-best-herbs-and-supplements-for-diabetes

Chapter 12

1. See more at http://www.diabetes.org/living-with-diabetes/treatment-and-care/blood-blucose-control/dawn-phenomenon.html

2. See more at http://mayoclinic.org/dawn-effect/

Made in United States
Troutdale, OR
11/03/2026

56844455R00115